1. Veggie omelet

Ingredient:

- 3 eggs
- 1/4 cup diced bell peppers
- 1/4 cup diced onions
- 1/4 cup diced mushrooms
- 1 tbsp olive oil
- Salt and pepper to taste

Instructions:

1. Crack the eggs into a bowl and beat them lightly with a fork. Season with a pinch of salt and pepper.

2. Heat the olive oil in a non•stick skillet over medium heat.

3. Add the diced bell peppers, onions, and mushrooms to the skillet. Sauté for 2•3 minutes until the vegetables are tender.

4. Pour the beaten eggs over the vegetables. Use a spatula to gently push the eggs from the edges into the center as they cook.

5. Once the bottom is set but the top is still a bit runny, fold the omelet in half and slide it onto a plate.

6. Serve hot and enjoy!

This veggie•packed omelet is a great high•protein, moderate•carb meal for endomorphs trying to manage their weight. The vegetables provide fiber and nutrients without too many carbs. Pair it with a small serving of whole grain toast or a side salad for a balanced endomorph•friendly breakfast or brunch.

Welcome to **"A Comprehensive Body,"** a guide designed to help you achieve your fitness goals through a holistic approach to health and wellness. This book is a comprehensive resource that combines muscle-building exercises with a carefully curated 30-day meal plan featuring over 110 delicious recipes for every meal of the day.

Whether you are a seasoned fitness enthusiast looking to take your workouts to the next level or a beginner seeking guidance on how to build muscle and improve your overall health, this book is tailored to meet your needs. By incorporating effective exercise plans and nutritious meal options, "A Comprehensive Body" aims to provide you with the tools and knowledge necessary to transform your body and enhance your well-being.

Throughout the pages of this book, you will find detailed workout routines, expert tips on maximizing your muscle-building potential, and a diverse array of recipes to fuel your body and support your fitness journey. From energizing breakfast options to satisfying dinner ideas and indulgent dessert recipes, each meal is carefully crafted to help you meet your nutritional needs while enjoying delicious and satisfying food.

Whether your goal is to increase muscle mass, improve your strength and endurance, or simply adopt a healthier lifestyle, "A Comprehensive Body" is your ultimate guide to achieving success. Get ready to embark on a transformative 30-day journey that will empower you to build a stronger, fitter, and healthier body from the inside out.

2. Scrambled eggs with spinach

Ingredient:

- 3 eggs
- 1 cup fresh spinach, chopped
- 1 tbsp olive oil
- 1 tbsp milk or unsweetened almond milk
- Salt and pepper to taste

Instructions:

1. Crack the eggs into a bowl and beat them lightly with a fork. Stir in the milk and season with a pinch of salt and pepper.

2. Heat the olive oil in a non•stick skillet over medium heat.

3. Add the chopped spinach to the skillet and sauté for 1•2 minutes until wilted.

4. Pour the egg mixture into the skillet with the spinach. Use a spatula to gently push the eggs from the edges into the center as they cook.

5. Continue cooking, stirring occasionally, until the eggs are softly scrambled and cooked through, about 2•3 minutes.

6. Remove from heat and serve immediately.

This scrambled egg dish is packed with protein from the eggs and nutrients from the spinach. The healthy fats from the olive oil help keep you feeling full. It's a great balanced meal for endomorphs that provides a good mix of protein, healthy fats, and moderate carbs from the spinach. Serve it with a small portion of whole grain toast or a side of roasted vegetables for a complete endomorph•friendly breakfast or brunch.

3. Egg muffins with veggies and turkey bacon

Ingredient:

- 6 eggs
- 1/2 cup diced bell peppers
- 1/4 cup diced onions
- 1/4 cup diced mushrooms
- 2 slices turkey bacon, cooked and crumbled
- 2 tbsp unsweetened almond milk
- Salt and pepper to taste

Instructions:

1. Preheat your oven to 350°F. Grease a 6•cup muffin tin with non•stick cooking spray.

2. In a medium bowl, whisk the eggs together with the almond milk. Season with a pinch of salt and pepper.

3. Stir in the diced bell peppers, onions, mushrooms, and crumbled turkey bacon.

4. Divide the egg mixture evenly among the 6 muffin cups.

5. Bake for 20•25 minutes, until the eggs are set and the tops are lightly golden.

6. Allow the egg muffins to cool for 5 minutes before removing them from the tin.

7. Serve warm and enjoy!

These egg muffins are a great make•ahead breakfast or snack option for endomorphs. The combination of protein•rich eggs, veggies, and turkey bacon provides a balanced meal that will help keep you feeling full and satisfied. The muffin format also makes them easy to grab and go. Pair these egg muffins with a piece of whole grain toast or a small serving of fresh fruit for a complete endomorph•friendly meal.

4. Greek yogurt with berries and nuts

Ingredient:

- 1 cup plain Greek yogurt
- 1/2 cup mixed berries (such as blueberries, raspberries, and blackberries)
- 2 tbsp chopped walnuts or almonds
- 1 tsp honey (optional)

Instructions:

1. In a parfait glass or bowl, layer half of the Greek yogurt.

2. Top the yogurt with half of the mixed berries.

3. Sprinkle half of the chopped nuts over the berries.

4. Repeat the layers, ending with the remaining yogurt, berries, and nuts.

5. If desired, drizzle the honey over the top.

This Greek yogurt parfait is a great endomorph•friendly breakfast or snack. The Greek yogurt provides protein to help keep you feeling full, while the berries add natural sweetness and fiber. The nuts contribute healthy fats and a satisfying crunch.

This parfait is a balanced combination of protein, complex carbs, and healthy fats • all important macronutrients for endomorphs trying to manage their weight and blood sugar levels. Feel free to adjust the portions to suit your individual needs.

5. Chia seed pudding

Ingredient:

- 1/4 cup chia seeds
- 1 cup unsweetened almond milk
- 1 tbsp honey (optional)
- 1/2 tsp vanilla extract
- 1/4 cup mixed berries (such as blueberries, raspberries, and blackberries)
- 1 tbsp chopped walnuts or almonds

Instructions:

1. In a medium bowl, whisk together the chia seeds, almond milk, honey (if using), and vanilla extract until well combined.

2. Cover the bowl and refrigerate for at least 2 hours, or overnight, stirring occasionally, until the chia seeds have thickened the mixture into a pudding•like consistency.

3. When ready to serve, divide the chia seed pudding into two bowls or jars.

4. Top each serving with 2 tbsp of the mixed berries and 1/2 tbsp of the chopped nuts.

This chia seed pudding is a nutrient•dense, endomorph•friendly breakfast or snack. The chia seeds provide protein, fiber, and healthy omega•3 fatty acids to help keep you feeling full and satisfied. The berries add natural sweetness and antioxidants, while the nuts contribute healthy fats and crunch.

You can adjust the sweetness by adding more or less honey to your taste. This recipe can also be made in advance and stored in the refrigerator for up to 4 days, making it a convenient and easy•to•prepare option for endomorphs.

6. Protein smoothie with greens

Ingredient:

- 1 cup unsweetened almond milk
- 1/2 cup plain Greek yogurt
- 1 scoop vanilla protein powder
- 1 cup packed spinach or kale
- 1/2 banana, frozen
- 1 tbsp almond butter
- 1 tsp honey (optional)

Instructions:

1. Add all the ingredients to a high•speed blender.

2. Blend on high speed until the mixture is smooth and creamy, about 1 minute.

3. Pour the smoothie into a glass and enjoy immediately.

This protein smoothie is a nutrient•dense and endomorph•friendly option for breakfast or a snack. The combination of Greek yogurt, protein powder, and almond butter provides a good amount of protein to help keep you feeling full. The greens add fiber, vitamins, and minerals, while the banana and honey (if using) provide natural sweetness.

The healthy fats from the almond butter and almond milk also help slow the absorption of the carbs, which is important for endomorphs who need to manage their blood sugar levels. You can adjust the sweetness by adding more or less honey to your taste.

This smoothie is easy to make and can be a convenient way for endomorphs to get a nutritious meal or snack on the go. Feel free to experiment with different greens, fruits, and nut butters to find your perfect endomorph•friendly smoothie combination.

7. Smoked salmon, cream cheese and cucumber

Ingredient:

- 4 oz smoked salmon, thinly sliced
- 2 oz cream cheese, softened
- 1 small cucumber, sliced into rounds
- 1 tbsp fresh dill, chopped (optional)
- Freshly ground black pepper

Instructions:

1. Spread about 1•2 tsp of cream cheese onto each cucumber round.

2. Top the cream cheese with a slice of smoked salmon.

3. Sprinkle the chopped dill (if using) and a pinch of black pepper over the top.

4. Serve immediately or refrigerate until ready to enjoy.

These smoked salmon, cream cheese, and cucumber bites make for a delicious and endomorph•friendly snack or appetizer. The combination of healthy fats from the salmon and cream cheese, along with the fiber and hydration from the cucumber, makes this a balanced and satisfying option for endomorphs.

The protein and healthy fats will help keep you feeling full, while the low•carb cucumber and lack of added sugars make this a great choice for managing blood sugar levels. The fresh dill adds a nice flavor boost, but is optional if you prefer a more simple preparation.

These bites can be made ahead of time and stored in the refrigerator for up to 3 days, making them a convenient and easy•to•grab snack option for endomorphs on the go. Adjust the portion sizes as needed to fit your individual dietary needs.

8. Cottage cheese with seeds and berries

Ingredient:

• 1 cup low•fat or full•fat cottage cheese
• 1/4 cup mixed berries (such as blueberries, raspberries, and blackberries)
• 1 tbsp chia seeds
• 1 tbsp pumpkin seeds
• 1 tsp honey (optional)

Instructions:

1. In a small bowl, combine the cottage cheese, mixed berries, chia seeds, and pumpkin seeds.

2. If desired, drizzle the honey over the top.

3. Stir gently to combine.

4. Enjoy immediately.

This cottage cheese snack is an excellent choice for endomorphs. The cottage cheese provides a good amount of protein to help keep you feeling full, while the berries add natural sweetness and fiber. The chia and pumpkin seeds contribute healthy fats, protein, and fiber as well.

The combination of protein, healthy fats, and complex carbs from the berries makes this a balanced snack that can help regulate blood sugar levels for endomorphs. The honey is optional, as the berries provide natural sweetness, but you can add a small drizzle if you prefer a slightly sweeter taste.

This snack can be enjoyed on its own or paired with a small serving of whole grain crackers or a handful of raw nuts for a more substantial endomorph•friendly meal. It's also easy to prepare in advance and store in the refrigerator for a quick and nutritious snack option.

9. Avocado egg salad

Ingredient:

- 4 hard•boiled eggs, chopped
- 1 ripe avocado, mashed
- 2 tbsp plain Greek yogurt
- 1 tbsp lemon juice
- 1 tbsp chopped fresh parsley
- 1/4 tsp garlic powder
- Salt and pepper to taste

Instructions:

1. In a medium bowl, combine the chopped hard•boiled eggs and mashed avocado.

2. Add the Greek yogurt, lemon juice, parsley, garlic powder, and a pinch of salt and pepper. Stir gently until well combined.

3. Taste and adjust seasoning as needed.

4. Serve the avocado egg salad on a bed of greens, with whole grain crackers, or stuffed into celery sticks.

This avocado egg salad is a nutrient•dense and endomorph•friendly option. The combination of protein•rich eggs and healthy fats from the avocado provides a filling and satisfying meal or snack. The Greek yogurt adds a creamy texture and a boost of protein, while the lemon juice and parsley provide fresh flavor.

This recipe is low in carbs and high in healthy fats and protein, making it an ideal choice for endomorphs who need to manage their blood sugar levels and keep their appetite under control. The avocado also provides fiber, which can help slow the absorption of carbs.

You can adjust the portion size to fit your individual needs, and serve it with a side of non•starchy vegetables for an even more balanced endomorph•friendly meal. This egg salad can be made in advance and stored in the refrigerator for up to 3 days.

10. Grilled chicken salad with vinaigrette

Ingredient:

For the Salad:
• 4 oz grilled chicken breast, sliced
• 2 cups mixed greens (such as spinach, arugula, and romaine)
• 1/2 cup diced cucumber
• 1/4 cup diced tomatoes
• 2 tbsp sliced almonds

For the Vinaigrette:
• 2 tbsp olive oil
• 1 tbsp balsamic vinegar
• 1 tsp Dijon mustard
• 1 tsp honey
• 1 garlic clove, minced
• Salt and pepper to taste

Instructions:

1. In a small bowl, whisk together all the vinaigrette ingredients until well combined. Set aside.

2. In a large salad bowl, combine the mixed greens, diced cucumber, diced tomatoes, and sliced almonds.

3. Top the salad with the grilled chicken slices.

4. Drizzle the vinaigrette over the salad and toss gently to coat. Serve immediately.

This grilled chicken salad with a balsamic vinaigrette is an excellent choice for endomorphs. The combination of lean protein from the chicken, healthy fats from the olive oil and almonds, and fiber•rich greens and vegetables makes it a well•balanced and nutrient•dense meal.

The vinaigrette dressing provides a flavorful, low•calorie way to dress the salad without adding too many carbs. The honey in the dressing adds a touch of sweetness, while the Dijon mustard and garlic provide a savory depth of flavor.

This salad is easy to prepare and can be customized to your liking. Feel free to add other endomorph•friendly toppings, such as avocado, hard•boiled eggs, or roasted bell peppers. Adjust the portion sizes as needed to fit your individual dietary needs.

11. Tuna salad lettuce wraps

Ingredient:

- 1 (5 oz) can of tuna, drained
- 2 tbsp plain Greek yogurt
- 1 tbsp Dijon mustard
- 1 tbsp diced celery
- 1 tbsp diced red onion
- 1 tsp lemon juice
- Salt and pepper to taste
- 4•6 large lettuce leaves (such as romaine or butter lettuce)

Instructions:

1. In a medium bowl, combine the drained tuna, Greek yogurt, Dijon mustard, diced celery, diced red onion, and lemon juice. Mix well until fully incorporated.

2. Season the tuna salad with salt and pepper to taste.

3. Lay the lettuce leaves flat on a plate or cutting board.

4. Scoop a portion of the tuna salad onto the center of each lettuce leaf.

5. Fold the sides of the lettuce leaf over the tuna salad and enjoy.

These tuna salad lettuce wraps are a great endomorph•friendly option. The tuna provides a good source of protein to help keep you feeling full, while the Greek yogurt adds creaminess without too many carbs. The vegetables provide fiber and nutrients without spiking your blood sugar.

The lettuce leaves act as a low•carb "wrap" to keep the tuna salad contained, making this a convenient and portable snack or light meal. You can adjust the amount of tuna salad per wrap depending on your individual needs and appetite.

This recipe is also easy to customize • you can add diced cucumber, bell peppers, or other veggies to the tuna salad, or try different types of lettuce leaves. Pair these tuna salad wraps with a side of fresh berries or a small serving of roasted nuts for a balanced endomorph•friendly meal.

12. Shrimp and avocado salad

Ingredient:

- 1 lb cooked shrimp, peeled and deveined
- 1 avocado, diced
- 1/2 cup diced cucumber
- 1/4 cup diced red onion
- 2 tbsp chopped fresh cilantro
- 2 tbsp olive oil
- 1 tbsp lime juice
- 1/4 tsp salt
- 1/4 tsp black pepper

Instructions:

1. In a large bowl, combine the cooked shrimp, diced avocado, cucumber, red onion, and chopped cilantro.

2. In a small bowl, whisk together the olive oil, lime juice, salt, and black pepper to make the dressing.

3. Pour the dressing over the shrimp and avocado mixture and gently toss to coat.

4. Serve immediately or refrigerate until ready to serve.

This shrimp and avocado salad is an excellent choice for endomorphs. The shrimp provides a lean source of protein to help keep you feeling full, while the avocado contributes healthy fats and fiber. The cucumber and red onion add crunch and flavor without too many carbs.

The simple olive oil and lime juice dressing complements the other ingredients without adding unnecessary sugars or carbs. You can adjust the amounts of each ingredient to suit your personal taste preferences and dietary needs.

This salad can be enjoyed on its own as a light meal or snack, or you can serve it over a bed of mixed greens for a more substantial endomorph•friendly lunch or dinner. It's also a great option for meal prepping, as it can be stored in the refrigerator for up to 3 days.

13. Salmon burgers with avocado

Ingredient:

- 1 lb wild•caught salmon, finely chopped or pulsed in a food processor
- 1 egg, beaten
- 2 tbsp almond flour
- 1 tbsp chopped fresh dill
- 1 tsp Dijon mustard
- 1/4 tsp salt
- 1/4 tsp black pepper
- 1 avocado, sliced
- 4 lettuce leaves or whole grain buns

Instructions:

1. In a medium bowl, combine the chopped salmon, beaten egg, almond flour, dill, Dijon mustard, salt, and pepper. Mix well until fully incorporated.

2. Divide the salmon mixture into 4 equal patties, about 1/2 inch thick.

3. Heat a large non•stick skillet over medium heat. Cook the salmon burgers for 3•4 minutes per side, or until lightly browned and cooked through.

4. Place each salmon burger on a lettuce leaf or whole grain bun. Top with sliced avocado.

5. Serve immediately and enjoy!

These salmon burgers are an excellent choice for endomorphs. Salmon is a great source of protein and healthy omega•3 fatty acids, which can help regulate blood sugar levels and keep you feeling full. The avocado adds more healthy fats and fiber to the meal.

The almond flour in the patties helps bind the burgers together without adding too many carbs. You can also serve the salmon burgers on a bed of greens or with a side of roasted vegetables for a complete endomorph•friendly meal.

This recipe is easy to prepare and can be made in advance. The salmon burgers can be stored in the refrigerator for up to 3 days or frozen for longer•term storage. Adjust the portion sizes as needed to fit your individual dietary needs.

14. Zucchini noodles with turkey meatballs

Ingredient:

For the Meatballs:
- 1 lb ground turkey
- 1/4 cup almond flour
- 1 egg
- 2 tbsp grated Parmesan cheese
- 1 tsp dried oregano
- 1/2 tsp garlic powder
- 1/4 tsp salt
- 1/4 tsp black pepper

For the Zucchini Noodles:
- 3 medium zucchinis, spiralized or julienned
- 1 tbsp olive oil
- 1 garlic clove, minced
- 1/4 tsp red pepper flakes (optional)
- Salt and pepper to taste

Instructions:

1. Preheat your oven to 400°F. Line a baking sheet with parchment paper.

2. In a medium bowl, combine all the meatball ingredients and mix well. Form the mixture into 12•14 small meatballs and place them on the prepared baking sheet.

3. Bake the meatballs for 18•20 minutes, or until cooked through.

4. While the meatballs are baking, heat the olive oil in a large skillet over medium heat. Add the minced garlic and sauté for 1 minute.

5. Add the spiralized or julienned zucchini noodles to the skillet. Sauté for 3•5 minutes, until the zucchini is tender but still has some bite.

6. Season the zucchini noodles with salt, pepper, and red pepper flakes (if using). Serve the zucchini noodles topped with the baked turkey meatballs.

This zucchini noodle and turkey meatball dish is an excellent choice for endomorphs. The zucchini noodles provide a low•carb, fiber•rich alternative to traditional pasta, while the turkey meatballs offer a lean source of protein to help keep you feeling full and satisfied.

The almond flour and Parmesan in the meatballs help bind them together without adding too many carbs. The simple seasoning of garlic, oregano, and pepper provides plenty of flavor without the need for high•carb sauces.

This meal is easy to prepare and can be made in advance for a quick and nutritious endomorph•friendly dinner. Adjust the portion sizes as needed to fit your individual dietary requirements. Serve with a side salad or additional roasted vegetables for a complete and balanced meal.

15. Spaghetti squash with bolognese sauce

Ingredient:

For the Bolognese Sauce:
• 1 lb ground turkey or lean ground beef
• 1 tbsp olive oil
• 1 onion, diced
• 2 garlic cloves, minced
• 1 (28 oz) can crushed tomatoes
• 2 tbsp tomato paste
• 1 tsp dried oregano
• 1/2 tsp dried basil
• 1/4 tsp red pepper flakes (optional)
• Salt and pepper to taste

For the Spaghetti Squash:
• 1 medium spaghetti squash, halved lengthwise and seeds removed
• 1 tbsp olive oil
• Salt and pepper to taste

Instructions:

1. Preheat your oven to 400°F. Line a baking sheet with parchment paper.

2. Place the spaghetti squash halves cut•side up on the prepared baking sheet. Drizzle with the olive oil and season with salt and pepper.

3. Roast the spaghetti squash for 40•50 minutes, or until tender when pierced with a fork.

4. While the spaghetti squash is roasting, prepare the bolognese sauce. In a large skillet, cook the ground turkey or beef over medium•high heat, breaking it up as it cooks, until browned, about 5•7 minutes.

5. Drain any excess fat from the skillet, then add the olive oil, diced onion, and minced garlic. Sauté for 2•3 minutes until the onion is translucent.

6. Stir in the crushed tomatoes, tomato paste, oregano, basil, and red pepper flakes (if using). Season with salt and pepper to taste.

7. Reduce the heat to low and let the bolognese sauce simmer for 10•15 minutes, stirring occasionally.

8. Once the spaghetti squash is cooked, use a fork to shred the flesh into spaghetti•like strands. Serve the spaghetti squash noodles topped with the bolognese sauce.

This spaghetti squash with bolognese sauce is an excellent endomorph•friendly meal. The spaghetti squash provides a low•carb, fiber•rich alternative to traditional pasta, while the bolognese sauce offers a hearty, protein•packed topping.

16. Cauliflower fried rice with chicken

Ingredient:

2 garlic cloves, minced
• 1 cup frozen peas and carrots
• 2 eggs, beaten
• 2 tbsp low•sodium soy sauce
or coconut aminos
• 1 tsp grated ginger
• Salt and pepper to taste

• 1 head of cauliflower, riced
(about 4 cups riced cauliflower)
• 1 tbsp sesame oil
• 1 lb boneless, skinless chicken
breasts, diced
• 1 onion, diced

Instructions:

1. In a large skillet or wok, heat the sesame oil over medium•high heat.

2. Add the diced chicken and sauté until cooked through, about 5•7 minutes. Remove the chicken from the skillet and set aside.

3. In the same skillet, sauté the diced onion for 2•3 minutes until translucent.

4. Add the minced garlic and riced cauliflower to the skillet. Sauté for 5•7 minutes, stirring frequently, until the cauliflower is tender.

5. Push the cauliflower mixture to the sides of the skillet, creating a well in the center. Pour the beaten eggs into the well and let them cook for 1•2 minutes, then scramble the eggs.

6. Once the eggs are cooked, mix them into the cauliflower mixture.

7. Add the cooked chicken, frozen peas and carrots, soy sauce or coconut aminos, and grated ginger to the skillet. Stir to combine and heat through.

8. Season with salt and pepper to taste. Serve the cauliflower fried rice with chicken immediately.

This cauliflower fried rice with chicken is an excellent choice for endomorphs. The riced cauliflower provides a low•carb alternative to traditional rice, while the chicken adds lean protein to help keep you feeling full and satisfied.

The addition of frozen peas and carrots provides fiber and nutrients without too many carbs. The soy sauce or coconut aminos add flavor without the need for high•carb sauces or seasonings.

17. Baked cod with roasted broccoli

Ingredient:

- 4 (6 oz) cod fillets
- 2 tbsp olive oil, divided
- 1 tsp garlic powder
- 1 tsp paprika
- Salt and pepper to taste
- 1 head of broccoli, cut into florets
- 1 tbsp lemon juice

Instructions:

1. Preheat your oven to 400°F. Line a baking sheet with parchment paper.

2. Place the cod fillets on the prepared baking sheet. Drizzle 1 tbsp of olive oil over the top and season with the garlic powder, paprika, salt, and pepper.

3. In a separate bowl, toss the broccoli florets with the remaining 1 tbsp of olive oil and season with salt and pepper.

4. Arrange the broccoli around the cod fillets on the baking sheet.

5. Bake for 15•20 minutes, or until the cod is cooked through and flakes easily with a fork, and the broccoli is tender and lightly browned.

6. Remove from the oven and drizzle the lemon juice over the cod. Serve the baked cod and roasted broccoli immediately.

This baked cod and roasted broccoli dish is an excellent choice for endomorphs. Cod is a lean, high•protein fish that is low in calories and carbs, making it a great option for managing blood sugar levels. The broccoli provides fiber, vitamins, and minerals without adding too many carbs.

The simple seasoning of garlic, paprika, salt, and pepper adds flavor without the need for high•carb sauces or marinades. The lemon juice at the end provides a fresh, bright note to the dish.

This meal is easy to prepare and can be made in advance for a quick and nutritious endomorph•friendly dinner. Adjust the portion sizes as needed to fit your individual dietary requirements. Serve with a small side of roasted vegetables or a salad for a complete and balanced meal.

18. Roasted pork tenderloin with Brussels sprouts

Ingredient:

- 1 lb pork tenderloin
- 1 tbsp olive oil
- 1 tsp garlic powder
- 1 tsp dried thyme
- 1/2 tsp salt
- 1/4 tsp black pepper
- 1 lb Brussels sprouts, trimmed and halved
- 2 tbsp olive oil
- 1 tbsp balsamic vinegar
- Salt and pepper to taste

Instructions:

1. Preheat your oven to 400°F. Line a baking sheet with parchment paper.

2. In a small bowl, combine the 1 tbsp of olive oil, garlic powder, dried thyme, 1/2 tsp of salt, and 1/4 tsp of black pepper. Rub this seasoning mixture all over the pork tenderloin.

3. Place the pork tenderloin on the prepared baking sheet.

4. In a separate bowl, toss the trimmed and halved Brussels sprouts with the 2 tbsp of olive oil, balsamic vinegar, and a pinch of salt and pepper.

5. Arrange the Brussels sprouts around the pork tenderloin on the baking sheet.

6. Roast the pork and Brussels sprouts for 25•30 minutes, or until the pork reaches an internal temperature of 145°F and the Brussels sprouts are tender and lightly browned.

7. Remove the pork tenderloin from the oven and let it rest for 5 minutes before slicing.

8. Serve the sliced pork tenderloin with the roasted Brussels sprouts.

This roasted pork tenderloin and Brussels sprouts dish is an excellent choice for endomorphs. Pork tenderloin is a lean, high•protein meat that is low in carbs, making it a great option for managing blood sugar levels. The Brussels sprouts provide fiber, vitamins, and minerals without adding too many carbs.

The simple seasoning of garlic, thyme, salt, and pepper adds flavor without the need for high•carb sauces or marinades. The balsamic vinegar in the Brussels sprouts provides a touch of sweetness to balance the savory flavors.

19. Beef and vegetable stir•fry

Ingredient:

- 1 lb flank steak, thinly sliced
- 2 tbsp coconut oil or avocado oil
- 1 red bell pepper, sliced
- 1 cup broccoli florets
- 1 cup sliced mushrooms
- 1 cup snow peas or snap peas
- 2 garlic cloves, minced
- 1 tbsp grated ginger
- 2 tbsp low•sodium soy sauce or coconut aminos
- 1 tsp sesame oil
- Salt and pepper to taste

Instructions:

1. Heat the coconut or avocado oil in a large skillet or wok over high heat.

2. Add the sliced flank steak and stir•fry for 2•3 minutes, until the beef is lightly browned. Remove the beef from the skillet and set aside.

3. Add the sliced bell pepper, broccoli florets, mushrooms, and snow/snap peas to the skillet. Stir•fry for 3•4 minutes, until the vegetables are crisp•tender.

4. Add the minced garlic and grated ginger to the skillet. Stir•fry for 1 minute, until fragrant.

5. Return the cooked beef to the skillet. Add the soy sauce or coconut aminos and sesame oil. Toss everything together and cook for an additional 1•2 minutes.

6. Season with salt and pepper to taste. Serve the beef and vegetable stir•fry immediately.

This beef and vegetable stir•fry is an excellent choice for endomorphs. The lean flank steak provides a good source of protein, while the variety of vegetables add fiber, vitamins, and minerals without too many carbs.

The stir•fry cooking method helps to retain the nutrients in the vegetables, and the simple seasoning of soy sauce or coconut aminos, garlic, and ginger adds flavor without the need for high•carb sauces.

This dish is easy to prepare and can be made in advance for a quick and nutritious endomorph•friendly meal. Adjust the portion sizes as needed to fit your individual dietary requirements. Serve over a bed of cauliflower rice or with a side of roasted nuts for a complete and balanced endomorph•friendly meal.

20. Chicken fajita lettuce wraps

Ingredient:

- 1 lb boneless, skinless chicken breasts, sliced into strips
- 1 tbsp olive oil
- 1 tsp chili powder
- 1 tsp cumin
- 1/2 tsp garlic powder
- 1/4 tsp salt
- 1/4 tsp black pepper
- 1 red bell pepper, sliced
- 1 green bell pepper, sliced
- 1 onion, sliced
- 8•10 large lettuce leaves (such as romaine or butter lettuce)
- Toppings (optional): avocado, salsa, sour cream, shredded cheese

Instructions:

1. In a large skillet or wok, heat the olive oil over medium•high heat.

2. Add the sliced chicken to the skillet and season with the chili powder, cumin, garlic powder, salt, and pepper. Sauté the chicken for 5•7 minutes, until cooked through.

3. Add the sliced bell peppers and onion to the skillet. Sauté for an additional 3•5 minutes, until the vegetables are tender•crisp.

4. Remove the skillet from the heat.

5. Lay the lettuce leaves flat on a plate or cutting board.

6. Scoop a portion of the chicken and vegetable mixture onto the center of each lettuce leaf.

7. Top the fajita filling with any desired toppings, such as avocado, salsa, sour cream, or shredded cheese. Fold the sides of the lettuce leaf over the filling and enjoy.

These chicken fajita lettuce wraps are an excellent choice for endomorphs. The lean chicken provides a good source of protein, while the bell peppers and onions add fiber and nutrients without too many carbs.

The simple seasoning of chili powder, cumin, and garlic provides plenty of flavor without the need for high•carb sauces or marinades. The lettuce leaves act as a low•carb "wrap" to keep the fajita filling contained.

You can customize the toppings to your liking, but be mindful of the carb content. Avocado, salsa, and sour cream are great options, while shredded cheese can be added in moderation.

21. Stuffed bell peppers with ground turkey

Ingredient:

- 4 medium bell peppers, halved lengthwise and seeds removed
- 1 lb ground turkey
- 1/2 cup cooked cauliflower rice
- 1/4 cup diced onion
- 2 garlic cloves, minced
- 1 tsp dried oregano
- 1/2 tsp paprika
- 1/4 tsp red pepper flakes (optional)
- Salt and pepper to taste
- 1/4 cup shredded mozzarella cheese (optional)

Instructions:

1. Preheat your oven to 375°F. Arrange the bell pepper halves in a baking dish or on a rimmed baking sheet.

2. In a large skillet, cook the ground turkey over medium•high heat, breaking it up as it cooks, until browned, about 5•7 minutes.

3. Drain any excess fat from the skillet, then add the cooked cauliflower rice, diced onion, minced garlic, oregano, paprika, and red pepper flakes (if using). Season with salt and pepper to taste. Stir to combine.

4. Spoon the turkey and vegetable mixture evenly into the bell pepper halves.

5. If using, sprinkle the shredded mozzarella cheese over the top of the stuffed peppers.

6. Bake the stuffed peppers for 25•30 minutes, or until the peppers are tender and the filling is hot. Serve the stuffed bell peppers immediately.

These stuffed bell peppers with ground turkey are an excellent choice for endomorphs. The bell peppers provide a low•carb "vessel" to hold the protein•rich turkey and vegetable filling. The cauliflower rice adds extra fiber and nutrients without too many carbs.

The simple seasoning of oregano, paprika, and optional red pepper flakes provides plenty of flavor without the need for high•carb sauces or toppings. The mozzarella cheese is optional, but it can add a nice creamy element to the dish.

22. Eggplant lasagna rolls

Ingredient:

- 2 tbsp tomato paste
- 1 tsp dried oregano
- 1/2 tsp dried basil
- Salt and pepper to taste
- 1 cup part•skim ricotta cheese
- 1/2 cup shredded mozzarella cheese
- 1 medium eggplant, sliced lengthwise into 8 thin slices
- 1 tbsp olive oil
- 1 lb ground turkey or lean ground beef
- 1 onion, diced
- 3 garlic cloves, minced
- 1 (28 oz) can crushed tomatoes

Instructions:

1. Preheat your oven to 375°F. Lightly grease a 9x13 inch baking dish.

2. Brush the eggplant slices lightly with olive oil and place them on a baking sheet. Roast the eggplant for 10•12 minutes, until tender and pliable.

3. In a large skillet, cook the ground turkey or beef over medium•high heat, breaking it up as it cooks, until browned, about 5•7 minutes. Drain any excess fat.

4. Add the diced onion and minced garlic to the skillet. Sauté for 2•3 minutes until the onion is translucent.

5. Stir in the crushed tomatoes, tomato paste, oregano, and basil. Season with salt and pepper to taste. Simmer the sauce for 10 minutes.

6. Spread 1/2 cup of the tomato sauce in the bottom of the prepared baking dish.

7. Place about 2•3 tbsp of the ricotta cheese onto the end of each roasted eggplant slice. Roll up the eggplant slices and place them seam•side down in the baking dish.

8. Pour the remaining tomato sauce over the eggplant rolls and sprinkle the shredded mozzarella cheese on top. Bake the eggplant lasagna rolls for 20•25 minutes, until the cheese is melted and bubbly. Serve hot and enjoy!

These eggplant lasagna rolls are an excellent choice for endomorphs. The eggplant provides a low•carb alternative to traditional lasagna noodles, while the ground turkey or beef offers a lean source of protein. The ricotta and mozzarella cheeses add creaminess without too many carbs.

The simple tomato sauce provides flavor without the need for high•carb ingredients. This dish is easy to prepare and can be made in advance for a quick and nutritious endomorph•friendly meal.

23. Seared scallops with asparagus

Ingredient:

- 1 lb sea scallops, patted dry
- 2 tbsp olive oil, divided
- 1 lb asparagus, trimmed and cut into 1·inch pieces
- 2 garlic cloves, minced
- 1 tbsp lemon juice
- 2 tbsp chopped fresh parsley
- Salt and pepper to taste

Instructions:

1. Heat 1 tbsp of olive oil in a large skillet over medium·high heat.

2. Season the scallops with salt and pepper. Sear the scallops for 2·3 minutes per side, until they develop a golden·brown crust. Transfer the seared scallops to a plate and set aside.

3. In the same skillet, heat the remaining 1 tbsp of olive oil over medium heat. Add the asparagus pieces and sauté for 3·4 minutes, until they are tender·crisp.

4. Add the minced garlic to the skillet and sauté for an additional 1 minute, until fragrant.

5. Return the seared scallops to the skillet with the asparagus and garlic. Drizzle the lemon juice over the top and sprinkle with the chopped fresh parsley.

6. Gently toss the scallops and asparagus to combine and heat through, about 2 minutes. Serve the seared scallops with asparagus immediately.

This seared scallops and asparagus dish is an excellent choice for endomorphs. Scallops are a lean, high·protein seafood that is low in carbs, making them a great option for managing blood sugar levels. The asparagus provides fiber, vitamins, and minerals without adding too many carbs.

The simple preparation of searing the scallops and sautéing the asparagus with garlic and lemon juice allows the natural flavors to shine without the need for high·carb sauces or seasonings.

This meal is easy to prepare and can be made in advance for a quick and nutritious endomorph·friendly dinner. Adjust the portion sizes as needed to fit your individual dietary requirements. Serve with a side of roasted vegetables or a small salad for a complete and balanced endomorph·friendly meal.

24. Slow cooker turkey chili

Ingredient:

- 1 lb ground turkey
- 1 onion, diced
- 3 garlic cloves, minced
- 2 bell peppers, diced
- 1 tsp oregano
- 1/2 tsp smoked paprika
- 1/4 tsp cayenne pepper (optional)
- Salt and pepper to taste

- 2 (15 oz) cans diced tomatoes
- 1 (15 oz) can tomato sauce
- 1 (15 oz) can kidney beans, rinsed and drained
- 1 (15 oz) can black beans, rinsed and drained
- 2 tbsp chili powder
- 1 tsp cumin

Instructions:

1. In a large skillet over medium•high heat, cook the ground turkey, breaking it up as it cooks, until browned, about 5•7 minutes. Drain any excess fat.

2. Transfer the cooked turkey to a slow cooker. Add the diced onion, minced garlic, and diced bell peppers. Stir to combine.

3. Pour in the diced tomatoes, tomato sauce, kidney beans, and black beans. Stir in the chili powder, cumin, oregano, smoked paprika, and cayenne pepper (if using).

4. Season with salt and pepper to taste.

5. Cover the slow cooker and cook on low for 6•8 hours or on high for 3•4 hours, until the flavors have melded and the chili has thickened.

6. Serve the turkey chili hot, garnished with any desired toppings such as avocado, shredded cheese, or chopped cilantro.

This slow cooker turkey chili is an excellent choice for endomorphs. The ground turkey provides a lean source of protein, while the beans and vegetables add fiber and complex carbs to help keep you feeling full and satisfied.

The combination of spices, including chili powder, cumin, and smoked paprika, adds plenty of flavor without the need for high•carb ingredients. The optional cayenne pepper provides a subtle heat, which can be adjusted to your preference.

This chili is easy to prepare and can be made in advance, making it a convenient and endomorph•friendly meal option. Adjust the portion sizes as needed to fit your individual dietary requirements. Serve with a side salad or roasted vegetables for a complete and balanced endomorph•friendly meal.

25. Grilled steak with chimichurri sauce

Ingredient:

For the Chimichurri Sauce:
- 1 cup fresh parsley, chopped
- 3 garlic cloves, minced
- 2 tbsp olive oil
- 1 tbsp red wine vinegar
- 1 tsp dried oregano
- 1/4 tsp red pepper flakes
- 1/4 tsp salt
- 1/4 tsp black pepper

For the Steak:
- 1 lb flank steak or skirt steak
- 1 tbsp olive oil
- Salt and pepper to taste

Instructions:

1. Make the chimichurri sauce: In a small bowl, combine the chopped parsley, minced garlic, olive oil, red wine vinegar, dried oregano, red pepper flakes, salt, and black pepper. Stir to mix well and set aside.

2. Pat the steak dry with paper towels and brush both sides with the 1 tbsp of olive oil. Season generously with salt and pepper.

3. Preheat your grill or grill pan to high heat.

4. Grill the steak for 3•5 minutes per side, depending on thickness, until it reaches your desired level of doneness. Transfer the grilled steak to a cutting board and let it rest for 5 minutes.

5. Slice the steak against the grain into thin strips. Serve the grilled steak immediately, drizzled with the chimichurri sauce.

This grilled steak with chimichurri sauce is an excellent choice for endomorphs. Flank or skirt steak are lean, high•protein cuts of meat that are low in carbs, making them a great option for managing blood sugar levels.

The chimichurri sauce, made with fresh parsley, garlic, olive oil, and vinegar, provides a flavorful and low•carb topping for the steak. The sauce is packed with healthy fats and antioxidants without the need for high•carb ingredients.

This meal is easy to prepare and can be made on the grill or in a grill pan for a quick and nutritious endomorph•friendly dinner. Adjust the portion sizes as needed to fit your individual dietary requirements. Serve with a side of roasted vegetables or a small salad for a complete and balanced endomorph•friendly meal.

26. Greek chicken kabobs with tzatziki

Ingredient:

For the Tzatziki Sauce:
• 1 cup plain Greek yogurt
• 1 cucumber, grated and squeezed dry
• 2 garlic cloves, minced
• 1 tbsp fresh lemon juice
• 1 tbsp chopped fresh dill
• 1/4 tsp salt

For the Chicken Kabobs:
• 1 lb boneless, skinless chicken breasts, cut into 1•inch cubes
• 1 red onion, cut into 1•inch pieces
• 1 red bell pepper, cut into 1•inch pieces
• 1 zucchini, cut into 1•inch pieces
• 2 tbsp olive oil
• 2 tsp dried oregano
• 1 tsp garlic powder
• 1/2 tsp salt
• 1/4 tsp black pepper

Instructions:

1. In a large bowl, combine the chicken, onion, bell pepper, and zucchini. Drizzle with the olive oil and sprinkle with the oregano, garlic powder, salt, and pepper. Toss to coat the ingredients evenly.

2. Thread the chicken and vegetables onto skewers, alternating the ingredients.

3. Preheat your grill or grill pan to medium•high heat.

4. Grill the chicken kabobs for 12•15 minutes, turning occasionally, until the chicken is cooked through and the vegetables are tender.

5. While the kabobs are grilling, make the tzatziki sauce. In a medium bowl, combine the Greek yogurt, grated cucumber, minced garlic, lemon juice, chopped dill, and salt. Stir to mix well. Serve the grilled chicken kabobs warm, with the tzatziki sauce on the side for dipping.

These Greek chicken kabobs with tzatziki sauce are an excellent choice for endomorphs. The lean chicken provides a good source of protein, while the vegetables add fiber and nutrients without too many carbs.

The simple seasoning of oregano, garlic, salt, and pepper provides plenty of flavor without the need for high•carb marinades or sauces. The tzatziki sauce, made with Greek yogurt, cucumber, and fresh herbs, adds a refreshing and creamy element to the dish without adding unnecessary carbs.

This recipe is easy to prepare and can be made on the grill or in the oven for a quick and nutritious endomorph•friendly meal. Adjust the portion sizes as needed to fit your individual dietary requirements. Serve with a side salad or roasted vegetables for a complete and balanced endomorph•friendly meal.

27. Taco salad with ground beef

Ingredient:

- 1 lb ground beef
- 1 packet taco seasoning
- 1 head romaine lettuce, chopped
- 1 cup cherry tomatoes, halved
- 1/2 cup shredded cheddar cheese
- 1/4 cup sliced black olives
- 1/4 cup diced red onion
- 1/4 cup plain Greek yogurt
- 2 tbsp salsa
- 1 tbsp lime juice
- Salt and pepper to taste

Instructions:

1. In a skillet over medium heat, cook the ground beef until browned and crumbled. Drain any excess fat. Stir in the taco seasoning and 2•3 tbsp water. Simmer for 5 minutes.

2. In a large salad bowl, combine the chopped romaine lettuce, cherry tomatoes, shredded cheddar, black olives, and red onion.

3. Top the salad with the seasoned ground beef.

4. In a small bowl, mix together the Greek yogurt, salsa, and lime juice to make the dressing.

5. Drizzle the dressing over the salad and toss gently to coat.

6. Season with salt and pepper to taste.

This taco salad is a great option for endomorphs as it's high in protein from the ground beef, contains healthy fats from the Greek yogurt dressing, and has plenty of fiber and nutrients from the vegetables. The portion sizes can be adjusted to fit your individual macros and calorie needs.

28. Buffalo chicken stuffed spaghetti squash

Ingredient:

- 1 medium spaghetti squash, halved lengthwise and seeds removed
- 1 lb boneless, skinless chicken breasts
- 1/2 cup buffalo sauce (such as Frank's RedHot)
- 1/2 cup shredded cheddar cheese
- 2 tbsp crumbled blue cheese (optional)
- 2 tbsp chopped green onions (optional)
- Salt and pepper to taste

Instructions:

1. Preheat oven to 400°F. Place the spaghetti squash halves cut·side down on a baking sheet. Bake for 30·40 minutes, until tender when pierced with a fork.

2. Meanwhile, place the chicken breasts in a pot and cover with water. Bring to a boil, then reduce heat and simmer for 15·20 minutes until cooked through. Shred the chicken using two forks.

3. In a bowl, mix the shredded chicken with the buffalo sauce until well coated.

4. Once the spaghetti squash is cooked, use a fork to gently scrape the flesh into strands, leaving a 1/2·inch border around the edges to create a "boat".

5. Stuff the spaghetti squash boats evenly with the buffalo chicken mixture.

6. Top each stuffed squash half with shredded cheddar cheese and crumbled blue cheese (if using).

7. Return the stuffed squash to the oven and bake for an additional 10·15 minutes, until the cheese is melted and bubbly.

8. Garnish with chopped green onions (if using) and serve immediately.

This dish is low in carbs, high in protein, and full of flavor from the buffalo chicken and melted cheese. It's a great keto·friendly or low·carb meal option.

29. Pesto zucchini noodles with chicken

Ingredient:

- 3•4 medium zucchinis, spiralized or julienned into noodles
- 1 boneless, skinless chicken breast, grilled and sliced
- 1/2 cup basil pesto (store•bought or homemade)
- 1/4 cup cherry tomatoes, halved
- 2 tbsp toasted pine nuts
- Grated parmesan cheese (optional)
- Salt and pepper to taste

Instructions:

1. Prepare the zucchini noodles by spiralizing or julienning the zucchinis. Set aside.

2. Grill or cook the chicken breast until cooked through. Slice or shred the chicken.

3. In a large bowl, toss the zucchini noodles with the basil pesto until the noodles are evenly coated.

4. Add the grilled chicken slices, cherry tomatoes, and toasted pine nuts. Toss gently to combine.

5. Season with salt and pepper to taste.

6. Serve immediately, garnished with grated parmesan cheese if desired.

The pesto coats the zucchini noodles beautifully, and the chicken adds protein to make this a complete and healthy meal. The cherry tomatoes and pine nuts provide nice texture and flavor contrasts. Enjoy!

30. Beef and broccoli

Ingredient:

- 1 lb flank steak, thinly sliced against the grain
- 3 cups broccoli florets
- 2 tbsp sesame oil
- 3 cloves garlic, minced
- 1 tbsp grated fresh ginger
- 1/4 cup low·sodium soy sauce
- 2 tbsp rice vinegar
- 1 tbsp Erythritol or other low·calorie sweetener
- 1 tsp sesame seeds
- Salt and pepper to taste

Instructions:

1. In a small bowl, whisk together the soy sauce, rice vinegar, and Erythritol. Set aside.

2. Heat the sesame oil in a large skillet or wok over high heat. Add the garlic and ginger and cook for 30 seconds, until fragrant.

3. Add the sliced beef to the pan and cook, stirring frequently, until the beef is browned and cooked through, about 3·5 minutes.

4. Add the broccoli florets to the pan and pour the soy sauce mixture over the top. Bring to a simmer and cook for 3·5 minutes, until the broccoli is tender·crisp.

5. Remove from heat and sprinkle with sesame seeds. Season with salt and pepper to taste.

6. Serve immediately, over cauliflower rice or zucchini noodles for a low·carb option.

This beef and broccoli dish is a great choice for endomorphs as it's high in protein from the beef, low in carbs, and contains healthy fats from the sesame oil. The broccoli provides fiber and nutrients. Adjust the portion sizes to fit your individual macros and calorie needs.

31. Curried chicken salad

Ingredient:

- 2 cups cooked, shredded chicken breast
- 1/2 cup plain Greek yogurt
- 2 tbsp mayonnaise
- 1 tsp curry powder
- 1/2 tsp ground cumin
- 1/4 tsp ground coriander
- 1/4 tsp garlic powder
- 1/4 tsp salt
- 1/8 tsp black pepper
- 1/2 cup diced celery
- 1/4 cup diced red onion
- 2 tbsp chopped cilantro (optional)
- 1 tbsp sliced almonds (optional)

Instructions:

1. In a large bowl, combine the shredded chicken, Greek yogurt, mayonnaise, curry powder, cumin, coriander, garlic powder, salt, and pepper. Mix well until fully incorporated.

2. Fold in the diced celery, red onion, and chopped cilantro (if using).

3. Taste and adjust seasoning as needed.

4. Serve the curried chicken salad on a bed of greens, stuffed in a tomato or avocado, or with whole grain crackers or sliced cucumber.

5. Garnish with sliced almonds (if using) just before serving.

This curried chicken salad is a great option for endomorphs as it's high in protein from the chicken, contains healthy fats from the yogurt and mayonnaise, and has fiber from the vegetables. The spices add flavor without adding extra calories or carbs. Adjust the portion sizes to fit your individual macros and calorie needs.

32. Baked salmon with lemon herb sauce

Ingredient:

For the Salmon:
- 4 (6 oz) salmon fillets
- 1 tbsp olive oil
- Salt and pepper to taste

For the Lemon Herb Sauce:
- 1/4 cup olive oil
- 2 tbsp lemon juice
- 2 tbsp chopped fresh parsley
- 1 tbsp chopped fresh dill
- 2 garlic cloves, minced
- 1/4 tsp salt
- 1/4 tsp black pepper

Instructions:

1. Preheat your oven to 400°F.
Line a baking sheet with parchment paper.

2. Place the salmon fillets on the prepared baking sheet. Drizzle the 1 tbsp of olive oil over the top and season with salt and pepper.

3. Bake the salmon for 12•15 minutes, or until it flakes easily with a fork and reaches an internal temperature of 145°F.

4. While the salmon is baking, make the lemon herb sauce. In a small bowl, whisk together the 1/4 cup of olive oil, lemon juice, chopped parsley, chopped dill, minced garlic, salt, and black pepper.

5. Once the salmon is cooked, transfer the fillets to a serving plate.

6. Drizzle the lemon herb sauce over the top of the baked salmon. Serve the salmon immediately, garnished with additional fresh herbs if desired.

This baked salmon with lemon herb sauce is an excellent choice for endomorphs. Salmon is a lean, high•protein fish that is low in carbs, making it a great option for managing blood sugar levels. The healthy fats in the salmon and olive oil also help keep you feeling full and satisfied.

The lemon herb sauce provides a flavorful and low•carb topping for the salmon, without the need for high•carb ingredients. The combination of fresh herbs, lemon, and garlic adds a bright and savory element to the dish.

This meal is easy to prepare and can be made in the oven for a quick and nutritious endomorph•friendly dinner. Adjust the portion sizes as needed to fit your individual dietary requirements. Serve with a side of roasted vegetables or a small salad for a complete and balanced endomorph•friendly meal.

33. Turkey meatloaf muffins

Ingredient:

- 1 lb ground turkey
- 1/2 cup almond flour
- 1/4 cup grated parmesan cheese
- 1 egg, beaten
- 1/4 cup diced onion
- 2 cloves garlic, minced
- 1 tsp dried oregano
- 1 tsp dried basil
- 1/2 tsp salt
- 1/4 tsp black pepper
- 1/4 cup sugar•free ketchup or tomato sauce

Instructions:

1. Preheat oven to 375°F. Grease a 12•cup muffin tin.

2. In a large bowl, combine the ground turkey, almond flour, parmesan cheese, beaten egg, onion, garlic, oregano, basil, salt, and pepper. Mix well until fully incorporated.

3. Divide the turkey mixture evenly among the 12 muffin cups, pressing it down gently to compact it.

4. Top each meatloaf muffin with about 1 tbsp of the sugar•free ketchup or tomato sauce.

5. Bake for 25•30 minutes, until the meatloaf is cooked through and the internal temperature reaches 165°F.

6. Allow the meatloaf muffins to cool for 5 minutes before removing them from the tin.

7. Serve warm, garnished with additional parsley or basil if desired.

These turkey meatloaf muffins are perfect for an endomorph diet. They are high in protein from the ground turkey, low in carbs thanks to the almond flour, and packed with flavor. The individual portions also make it easy to control your serving size. Adjust the recipe as needed to fit your macros.

34. Cauliflower pizza with prosciutto

Ingredient:

For the Cauliflower Crust:
• 1 head of cauliflower, riced (about 4 cups riced)
• 1 egg, beaten
• 1/2 cup shredded mozzarella cheese
• 2 tbsp grated parmesan cheese
• 1 tsp dried oregano
• 1/2 tsp garlic powder
• 1/4 tsp salt

Toppings:
• 1/2 cup marinara or pizza sauce
• 8 oz shredded mozzarella cheese
• 4 oz thinly sliced prosciutto
• 1/4 cup grated parmesan cheese
• Fresh basil leaves (optional)

Instructions:

1. Preheat oven to 400°F. Line a baking sheet with parchment paper.

2. To make the cauliflower crust, place the riced cauliflower in a microwave•safe bowl and microwave for 5•7 minutes, until tender. Allow to cool slightly.

3. Transfer the cauliflower to a clean kitchen towel and squeeze out as much moisture as possible.

4. In a bowl, mix the squeezed cauliflower, beaten egg, mozzarella, parmesan, oregano, garlic powder, and salt until well combined.

5. Press the cauliflower mixture onto the prepared baking sheet, forming a round pizza crust about 1/4•inch thick.

6. Bake the crust for 20•25 minutes, until golden brown.

7. Remove the crust from the oven and top with the marinara sauce, shredded mozzarella, prosciutto slices, and grated parmesan.

8. Return the pizza to the oven and bake for an additional 10•15 minutes, until the cheese is melted and bubbly. Remove from oven, garnish with fresh basil leaves (if using), and slice to serve.

This cauliflower pizza is a great low•carb option for an endomorph diet. The cauliflower crust provides fiber, while the prosciutto and cheese add protein and healthy fats. Adjust the portion sizes as needed to fit your individual macros.

35. Blackened fish tacos with slaw

Ingredient:

For the Fish:
• 1 lb white fish fillets
(such as tilapia, cod, or mahi•mahi)
• 2 tsp chili powder
• 1 tsp smoked paprika
• 1 tsp garlic powder
• 1/2 tsp onion powder
• 1/2 tsp cumin
• 1/4 tsp cayenne pepper
• Salt and pepper to taste

For the Slaw:
• 2 cups shredded cabbage (green and/or red)
• 1/4 cup plain Greek yogurt
• 2 tbsp lime juice
• 1 tsp honey
• 1/4 tsp salt

For Serving:
• 8•10 small corn or flour tortillas
• Diced avocado
• Chopped cilantro
• Lime wedges

Instructions:

1. In a small bowl, mix together the chili powder, paprika, garlic powder, onion powder, cumin, and cayenne. Season the fish fillets generously with the spice mixture on both sides.

2. In a large skillet over medium•high heat, cook the blackened fish fillets for 3•4 minutes per side, until cooked through and flaky.

3. In a medium bowl, combine the shredded cabbage, Greek yogurt, lime juice, honey, and salt. Toss to coat the slaw.

4. Warm the tortillas according to package instructions.

5. Flake the blackened fish into chunks and divide evenly among the tortillas. Top each taco with the slaw, diced avocado, and chopped cilantro. Serve immediately with lime wedges.

These blackened fish tacos are a great option for an endomorph diet. The fish provides lean protein, the slaw adds fiber and nutrients, and the whole meal is low in carbs. Adjust the portion sizes as needed to fit your individual macros.

36. Asian chicken lettuce wraps

Ingredient:

- 1 lb ground chicken or turkey
- 2 tbsp sesame oil
- 3 cloves garlic, minced
- 1 tbsp grated fresh ginger
- 2 tbsp low•sodium soy sauce
- 1 tbsp rice vinegar
- 1 tsp Erythritol or other low•calorie sweetener
- 1/4 tsp red pepper flakes (optional)
- 1 cup shredded cabbage or coleslaw mix
- 1/2 cup diced water chestnuts
- 2 tbsp chopped green onions
- 1 head of butter or romaine lettuce, leaves separated

Instructions:

1. In a large skillet or wok, heat the sesame oil over medium•high heat. Add the ground chicken and cook, breaking it up with a spatula, until browned and cooked through, about 5•7 minutes.

2. Add the garlic and ginger to the pan and cook for 1 minute, until fragrant.

3. In a small bowl, whisk together the soy sauce, rice vinegar, and Erythritol. Pour the sauce into the pan with the chicken and stir to combine.

4. Stir in the shredded cabbage, water chestnuts, and green onions. Cook for 2•3 minutes, until the cabbage is slightly wilted.

5. Serve the chicken mixture in the lettuce leaves, allowing guests to assemble their own wraps.

6. Optionally, top with additional green onions, toasted sesame seeds, or a drizzle of sriracha or other hot sauce.

This Asian•inspired chicken lettuce wrap recipe is perfect for an endomorph diet. It's low in carbs, high in protein, and packed with flavor from the soy sauce, ginger, and garlic. The crunchy cabbage and water chestnuts add great texture. Adjust the portion sizes as needed to fit your individual macros.

37. Sausage and peppers

Ingredient:

- 1 lb Italian sausage links, cut into 1-inch pieces
- 2 tbsp olive oil
- 1 large onion, sliced
- 3 bell peppers (mix of colors), sliced
- 3 cloves garlic, minced
- 1 tsp dried oregano
- 1/2 tsp red pepper flakes (optional)
- 1/4 cup low-sodium chicken broth
- Salt and pepper to taste

Instructions:

1. In a large skillet or Dutch oven, heat the olive oil over medium-high heat. Add the sausage pieces and cook, stirring occasionally, until browned on all sides, about 5-7 minutes. Transfer the sausage to a plate and set aside.

2. Add the sliced onions to the same pan and cook for 3-4 minutes, until starting to soften.

3. Add the sliced bell peppers and continue cooking for 5-7 minutes, until the peppers are tender-crisp.

4. Stir in the minced garlic, oregano, and red pepper flakes (if using). Cook for 1 minute, until fragrant.

5. Pour in the chicken broth and use a wooden spoon to scrape up any browned bits from the bottom of the pan.

6. Return the cooked sausage to the pan and simmer for 5-10 minutes, until the sauce has thickened slightly.

7. Season with salt and pepper to taste.

8. Serve the sausage and peppers over zucchini noodles, cauliflower rice, or on their own.

This sausage and peppers dish is a great option for an endomorph diet. It's high in protein from the sausage, low in carbs, and packed with fiber and nutrients from the peppers and onions. Adjust the portion sizes as needed to fit your individual macros.

38. Chicken cacciatore over zucchini noodles

Ingredient:

- 1 lb boneless, skinless chicken thighs, cut into 1•inch pieces
- 2 tbsp olive oil
- 1 onion, diced
- 3 cloves garlic, minced
- 1 cup sliced mushrooms
- 1 red bell pepper, diced
- 1 (14.5 oz) can diced tomatoes
- 1/2 cup dry red wine (or low•sodium chicken broth)
- 1 tsp dried oregano
- 1/2 tsp dried thyme
- 1/4 tsp red pepper flakes (optional)
- Salt and pepper to taste
- 3•4 medium zucchinis, spiralized or julienned into noodles

Instructions:

1. In a large skillet or Dutch oven, heat the olive oil over medium•high heat. Add the chicken pieces and cook, stirring occasionally, until browned on all sides, about 5•7 minutes. Transfer the chicken to a plate and set aside.

2. Add the diced onion to the same pan and cook for 3•4 minutes, until translucent. Add the minced garlic and cook for 1 minute more.

3. Stir in the sliced mushrooms and diced bell pepper. Cook for 5 minutes, until the vegetables are tender.

4. Pour in the diced tomatoes with their juices and the red wine (or chicken broth). Add the dried oregano, thyme, and red pepper flakes (if using). Season with salt and pepper.

5. Return the browned chicken to the pan and bring the mixture to a simmer. Reduce heat to medium•low and let the cacciatore simmer for 15•20 minutes, until the chicken is cooked through and the sauce has thickened.

6. While the cacciatore is simmering, prepare the zucchini noodles. Serve the chicken cacciatore over the zucchini noodles.

This chicken cacciatore dish is a great low•carb option for an endomorph diet. The zucchini noodles provide a healthy, veggie•based alternative to pasta, while the chicken and vegetables offer protein, fiber, and nutrients. Adjust the portion sizes as needed to fit your individual macros.

39. Grilled shrimp skewers

Ingredient:

- 1 lb large shrimp, peeled and deveined
- 2 tbsp olive oil
- 2 tbsp lemon juice
- 2 cloves garlic, minced
- 1 tsp dried oregano
- 1/2 tsp paprika
- 1/4 tsp red pepper flakes (optional)
- Salt and pepper to taste
- Lemon wedges for serving

Instructions:

1. In a large bowl, combine the shrimp, olive oil, lemon juice, garlic, oregano, paprika, and red pepper flakes (if using). Toss to coat the shrimp evenly. Season with salt and pepper.

2. Thread the marinated shrimp onto metal or wooden skewers, leaving a little space between each shrimp.

3. Preheat your grill or grill pan to medium·high heat.

4. Grill the shrimp skewers for 2·3 minutes per side, until the shrimp are opaque and cooked through.

5. Serve the grilled shrimp skewers immediately, with lemon wedges on the side.

Optional Serving Suggestions:
- Serve the shrimp skewers over a bed of zucchini noodles or cauliflower rice for a low·carb meal.
- Pair the shrimp with a fresh salad or roasted vegetables.
- Sprinkle with chopped fresh parsley or cilantro for extra flavor.

These grilled shrimp skewers are a great option for an endomorph diet. Shrimp is a lean protein, and the marinade adds flavor without adding many calories or carbs. Adjust the portion sizes as needed to fit your individual macros and calorie needs.

40. Lamb meatballs with mint yogurt sauce

Ingredient:

For the Meatballs:
• 1 lb ground lamb
• 1/4 cup almond flour
• 1 egg, beaten
• 2 cloves garlic, minced
• 1 tsp ground cumin
• 1 tsp dried oregano
• 1/2 tsp salt
• 1/4 tsp black pepper

For the Mint Yogurt Sauce:
• 1 cup plain Greek yogurt
• 2 tbsp chopped fresh mint
• 1 tbsp lemon juice
• 1 clove garlic, minced
• 1/4 tsp salt

Instructions:

1. Preheat oven to 400°F. Line a baking sheet with parchment paper.

2. In a large bowl, combine all the meatball ingredients and mix well until fully incorporated. Roll the mixture into 1•inch meatballs and place them on the prepared baking sheet.

3. Bake the meatballs for 18•20 minutes, until cooked through and lightly browned.

4. While the meatballs are baking, make the mint yogurt sauce. In a small bowl, mix together the Greek yogurt, chopped mint, lemon juice, minced garlic, and salt. Stir until well combined. Serve the warm lamb meatballs with the mint yogurt sauce on the side for dipping.

Optional Serving Suggestions:
• Serve the meatballs and sauce over a bed of cauliflower rice or zucchini noodles for a low•carb meal.
• Garnish with additional chopped mint and a sprinkle of lemon zest.
• Offer the meatballs as an appetizer or snack.

These lamb meatballs are a great option for an endomorph diet. The lamb provides high•quality protein, while the almond flour and yogurt sauce keep the dish low in carbs. Adjust the portion sizes as needed to fit your individual macros.

41. Beef and cabbage stir•fry

Ingredient:

- 1 lb beef sirloin or flank steak, thinly sliced
- 2 tbsp sesame oil
- 3 cloves garlic, minced
- 1 tbsp grated fresh ginger
- 1/2 head green cabbage, thinly sliced (about 4 cups)
- 1 red bell pepper, thinly sliced
- 2 tbsp low•sodium soy sauce
- 1 tbsp rice vinegar
- 1 tsp Erythritol or other low•calorie sweetener
- 1/4 tsp red pepper flakes (optional)
- Salt and pepper to taste
- Chopped green onions and sesame seeds for garnish (optional)

Instructions:

1. In a large skillet or wok, heat the sesame oil over high heat.

2. Add the sliced beef and cook, stirring frequently, until browned and cooked through, about 3•5 minutes. Transfer the beef to a plate and set aside.

3. Add the minced garlic and grated ginger to the same pan and cook for 1 minute, until fragrant.

4. Add the sliced cabbage and bell pepper to the pan. Stir•fry for 3•5 minutes, until the vegetables are tender•crisp.

5. Return the cooked beef to the pan and add the soy sauce, rice vinegar, Erythritol, and red pepper flakes (if using). Toss everything together and cook for 2•3 minutes, until heated through.

6. Season with salt and pepper to taste. Serve the beef and cabbage stir•fry immediately, garnished with chopped green onions and sesame seeds if desired.

This beef and cabbage stir•fry is a great option for an endomorph diet. It's high in protein from the beef, low in carbs, and packed with fiber and nutrients from the vegetables. Adjust the portion sizes as needed to fit your individual macros.

42. Sesame•ginger baked tofu

Ingredient:
- 1 block (14 oz) extra•firm tofu, pressed and cut into 1•inch cubes
- 2 tbsp low•sodium soy sauce
- 1 tbsp rice vinegar
- 1 tbsp sesame oil
- 1 tbsp grated fresh ginger
- 1 tsp Erythritol or other low•calorie sweetener
- 1/4 tsp red pepper flakes (optional)
- 1 tbsp sesame seeds
- 2 tsp olive oil
- Salt and pepper to taste

Instructions:
1. Preheat your oven to 400°F. Line a baking sheet with parchment paper.

2. In a medium bowl, whisk together the soy sauce, rice vinegar, sesame oil, grated ginger, Erythritol, and red pepper flakes (if using).

3. Add the tofu cubes to the bowl and gently toss to coat them evenly in the marinade.

4. Spread the marinated tofu cubes in a single layer on the prepared baking sheet. Sprinkle the sesame seeds over the top.

5. Drizzle the olive oil over the tofu.

6. Bake for 20•25 minutes, flipping the tofu cubes halfway through, until they are golden brown and crispy. Remove the baked tofu from the oven and season with salt and pepper to taste.

Serving Suggestions:
- Serve the sesame•ginger baked tofu over a bed of steamed broccoli or cauliflower rice for a complete low•carb meal.
- Toss the tofu with a stir•fried vegetable medley.
- Use the baked tofu cubes as a protein•rich snack or addition to salads.

This sesame•ginger baked tofu is a great option for an endomorph diet. The tofu provides plant•based protein, while the marinade adds flavor without adding many carbs. Adjust the portion sizes as needed to fit your individual macros.

43. Pork carnitas lettuce cups

Ingredient:

• 2 lbs boneless pork shoulder, cut into 2•inch cubes
• 1 onion, diced
• 4 cloves garlic, minced
• 1 tbsp cumin
• 1 tsp oregano
• 1 tsp chili powder
• 1/2 tsp smoked paprika
• 1/4 tsp cayenne pepper (optional)
• 1 cup low•sodium chicken or beef broth
• 2 tbsp lime juice
• Salt and pepper to taste
• 1 head of romaine or butter lettuce, leaves separated

For Serving:
• Diced avocado
• Chopped cilantro
• Lime wedges

Instructions:

1. In a large slow cooker or Dutch oven, combine the pork cubes, diced onion, minced garlic, cumin, oregano, chili powder, smoked paprika, and cayenne (if using). Season with salt and pepper.

2. Pour in the broth and lime juice. Stir to combine.

3. If using a slow cooker, cook on low for 7•8 hours or on high for 4•5 hours, until the pork is very tender and shreds easily.

4. If using a Dutch oven, bring the mixture to a boil, then reduce heat to low, cover, and simmer for 2•3 hours, until the pork is tender.

5. Once the pork is cooked, use two forks to shred it directly in the slow cooker or Dutch oven. Serve the shredded pork carnitas in the lettuce cups, topped with diced avocado, chopped cilantro, and a squeeze of fresh lime juice.

This pork carnitas lettuce cup recipe is perfect for an endomorph diet. The pork provides protein, the lettuce cups are low in carbs, and the toppings add healthy fats and nutrients. Adjust the portion sizes as needed to fit your individual macros.

44. Moroccan chicken stew

Ingredient:

- 1/4 tsp cayenne pepper (optional)
- 1 (14.5 oz) can diced tomatoes
- 1 cup low•sodium chicken broth
- 1 cup cauliflower florets
- 1 cup diced zucchini
- 1/4 cup sliced green olives
- 2 tbsp chopped fresh cilantro
- Salt and pepper to taste

- 1 lb boneless, skinless chicken thighs, cut into 1•inch pieces
- 2 tbsp olive oil
- 1 onion, diced
- 3 cloves garlic, minced
- 1 tbsp grated fresh ginger
- 1 tsp ground cumin
- 1 tsp ground coriander
- 1 tsp paprika
- 1/2 tsp ground cinnamon

Instructions:

1. In a large pot or Dutch oven, heat the olive oil over medium•high heat. Add the chicken pieces and cook, stirring occasionally, until browned on all sides, about 5•7 minutes. Transfer the chicken to a plate and set aside.

2. Add the diced onion to the same pot and cook for 3•4 minutes, until translucent. Add the minced garlic and grated ginger and cook for 1 minute more.

3. Stir in the cumin, coriander, paprika, cinnamon, and cayenne (if using). Cook for 1 minute, until fragrant.

4. Pour in the diced tomatoes with their juices and the chicken broth. Bring the mixture to a simmer.

5. Add the cauliflower florets, diced zucchini, and the cooked chicken back to the pot. Simmer for 15•20 minutes, until the vegetables are tender and the chicken is cooked through.

6. Stir in the sliced green olives and chopped cilantro. Season with salt and pepper to taste. Serve the Moroccan chicken stew warm, garnished with additional cilantro if desired.

This Moroccan chicken stew is a great option for an endomorph diet. It's high in protein from the chicken, low in carbs, and packed with fiber and nutrients from the vegetables. Adjust the portion sizes as needed to fit your individual macros.

45. Garlic shrimp with zucchini noodles

Ingredient:

- 1 lb large shrimp, peeled and deveined
- 2 tbsp olive oil
- 4 cloves garlic, minced
- 1/4 tsp red pepper flakes (optional)
- 1/4 cup dry white wine or low•sodium chicken broth
- 2 tbsp lemon juice
- 2 tbsp chopped fresh parsley
- Salt and pepper to taste
- 3•4 medium zucchinis, spiralized or julienned into noodles

Instructions:

1. In a large skillet, heat the olive oil over medium•high heat.

2. Add the minced garlic and red pepper flakes (if using) to the hot oil. Cook for 1 minute, stirring constantly, until fragrant.

3. Add the shrimp to the skillet and cook for 2•3 minutes per side, until the shrimp are opaque and cooked through.

4. Pour in the white wine (or chicken broth) and lemon juice. Bring the mixture to a simmer and cook for 2•3 minutes, allowing the sauce to thicken slightly.

5. Remove the skillet from heat and stir in the chopped parsley. Season with salt and pepper to taste.

6. Add the spiralized or julienned zucchini noodles to the skillet and toss to coat them in the garlic•shrimp sauce. Serve the garlic shrimp and zucchini noodles immediately.

Optional Serving Suggestions:
- Top with grated parmesan cheese or crumbled feta.
- Garnish with additional chopped parsley or lemon wedges.
- Serve with a side salad for a complete low•carb meal.

This garlic shrimp with zucchini noodles dish is a great option for an endomorph diet. The shrimp provides protein, the zucchini noodles are low in carbs, and the dish is full of flavor from the garlic, lemon, and parsley. Adjust the portion sizes as needed to fit your individual macros.

46. Italian sausage and kale soup

Ingredient:

• 1 lb Italian sausage, casings removed
• 1 onion, diced
• 3 cloves garlic, minced
• 4 cups low•sodium chicken broth
• 1 (14.5 oz) can diced tomatoes
• 1 tsp dried oregano
• 1/2 tsp dried basil
• 1/4 tsp red pepper flakes (optional)
• 4 cups chopped kale, stems removed
• 1 cup sliced mushrooms
• 1/4 cup grated parmesan cheese (optional)
• Salt and pepper to taste

Instructions:

1. In a large pot or Dutch oven, cook the Italian sausage over medium•high heat, breaking it up with a wooden spoon, until browned and cooked through, about 5•7 minutes. Transfer the sausage to a plate and set aside.

2. Add the diced onion to the same pot and cook for 3•4 minutes, until translucent. Add the minced garlic and cook for 1 minute more.

3. Pour in the chicken broth and diced tomatoes with their juices. Stir in the dried oregano, basil, and red pepper flakes (if using).

4. Bring the soup to a simmer, then add the cooked sausage, chopped kale, and sliced mushrooms. Simmer for 10•15 minutes, until the kale is tender.

5. Remove the soup from heat and stir in the grated parmesan cheese, if using.

6. Season the soup with salt and pepper to taste.

7. Serve the Italian sausage and kale soup hot, garnished with additional parmesan cheese if desired.

This hearty soup is a great option for an endomorph diet. The Italian sausage provides protein, the kale and mushrooms add fiber and nutrients, and the overall dish is low in carbs. Adjust the portion sizes as needed to fit your individual macros.

47. Cajun cod with roasted okra

Ingredient:

For the Okra:
- 1 lb fresh okra, trimmed and halved lengthwise
- 2 tbsp olive oil
- 1 tsp Cajun seasoning
- Salt and pepper to taste

For the Cod:
- 4 (6 oz) cod fillets
- 2 tbsp Cajun seasoning
- 1 tbsp olive oil

Instructions:

1. Preheat your oven to 400°F. Line a baking sheet with parchment paper.

2. In a large bowl, toss the halved okra with the olive oil, Cajun seasoning, salt, and pepper until evenly coated.

3. Spread the okra in a single layer on the prepared baking sheet. Roast for 15•20 minutes, tossing halfway, until the okra is tender and lightly browned.

4. While the okra is roasting, pat the cod fillets dry and season both sides generously with the Cajun seasoning.

5. Heat the 1 tbsp of olive oil in a large skillet over medium•high heat.

6. Add the seasoned cod fillets to the hot skillet and cook for 3•4 minutes per side, until the fish is opaque and flakes easily with a fork. Serve the Cajun cod immediately, topped with the roasted okra.

Optional Serving Suggestions:
- Serve the cod and okra over a bed of cauliflower rice or zucchini noodles for a low•carb meal.
- Garnish with chopped fresh parsley or green onions.
- Squeeze a little lemon juice over the top before serving.

This Cajun cod with roasted okra dish is a great option for an endomorph diet. The cod provides lean protein, the okra adds fiber and nutrients, and the Cajun seasoning adds tons of flavor without many carbs. Adjust the portion sizes as needed to fit your individual macros.

48. Broccoli beef

Ingredient:
- 1 lb flank steak, thinly sliced against the grain
- 2 tbsp sesame oil
- 3 cups broccoli florets
- 2 cloves garlic, minced
- 1 tbsp grated fresh ginger
- 2 tbsp low•sodium soy sauce
- 1 tbsp rice vinegar
- 1 tsp Erythritol or other low•calorie sweetener
- 1/4 tsp red pepper flakes (optional)
- Salt and pepper to taste
- Sesame seeds for garnish (optional)

Instructions:

1. In a large skillet or wok, heat the sesame oil over high heat.

2. Add the sliced beef to the hot pan and cook, stirring frequently, until browned and cooked through, about 3•5 minutes. Transfer the beef to a plate and set aside.

3. Add the broccoli florets to the same pan and stir•fry for 2•3 minutes, until the broccoli is tender•crisp.

4. Push the broccoli to the sides of the pan and add the minced garlic and grated ginger to the center. Cook for 1 minute, until fragrant.

5. Return the cooked beef to the pan and add the soy sauce, rice vinegar, Erythritol, and red pepper flakes (if using). Toss everything together and cook for 2•3 minutes, until heated through.

6. Season with salt and pepper to taste.

7. Serve the broccoli beef immediately, garnished with sesame seeds if desired.

This broccoli beef dish is a great option for an endomorph diet. The beef provides protein, the broccoli adds fiber and nutrients, and the dish is low in carbs. Adjust the portion sizes as needed to fit your individual macros.

49. Chicken piccata with cauliflower rice

Ingredient:

For the Cauliflower Rice:
• 1 head of cauliflower, riced
• 1 tbsp olive oil
• 1 clove garlic, minced
• Salt and pepper to taste

For the Chicken Piccata:
• 4 boneless, skinless chicken breasts, pounded thin
• 2 tbsp olive oil
• 2 tbsp lemon juice
• 2 tbsp capers, drained
• 1/4 cup dry white wine or low•sodium chicken broth
• 2 tbsp unsalted butter
• 2 tbsp chopped fresh parsley
• Salt and pepper to taste

Instructions:

1. In a large skillet, heat the 2 tbsp of olive oil over medium•high heat.

2. Season the pounded chicken breasts with salt and pepper on both sides. Add the chicken to the hot skillet and cook for 3•4 minutes per side, until golden brown and cooked through. Transfer the chicken to a plate and set aside.

3. In the same skillet, add the lemon juice, capers, and white wine (or chicken broth). Bring the mixture to a simmer, scraping up any browned bits from the bottom of the pan.

4. Reduce the heat to low and whisk in the 2 tbsp of unsalted butter until the sauce is smooth and creamy.

5. Return the cooked chicken to the skillet and spoon the sauce over the top. Sprinkle with chopped parsley.

6. In a separate skillet, heat the 1 tbsp of olive oil over medium heat. Add the riced cauliflower and minced garlic. Cook for 5•7 minutes, stirring occasionally, until the cauliflower is tender.

7. Season the cauliflower rice with salt and pepper to taste. Serve the chicken piccata immediately, over the cauliflower rice.

This chicken piccata dish is a great low•carb option for an endomorph diet. The chicken provides protein, the cauliflower rice is a healthy alternative to traditional rice, and the lemon•caper sauce adds tons of flavor. Adjust the portion sizes as needed to fit your individual macros.

50. Baked Italian meatballs

Ingredient:

• 1 lb ground beef
• 1 lb ground Italian sausage
• 1 cup almond flour
• 1/2 cup grated parmesan cheese
• 2 eggs, beaten
• 3 cloves garlic, minced
• 1 tsp dried oregano
• 1 tsp dried basil
• 1/2 tsp red pepper flakes (optional)
• 1/2 tsp salt
• 1/4 tsp black pepper

Instructions:

1. Preheat your oven to 400°F. Line a baking sheet with parchment paper.

2. In a large bowl, combine the ground beef, ground Italian sausage, almond flour, parmesan cheese, beaten eggs, minced garlic, oregano, basil, red pepper flakes (if using), salt, and pepper. Mix well until fully incorporated.

3. Scoop the meatball mixture by the tablespoon and roll into 1•inch balls, placing them on the prepared baking sheet.

4. Bake the meatballs for 18•22 minutes, until they are cooked through and lightly browned.

Serving Suggestions:
• Serve the baked meatballs over a bed of zucchini noodles or cauliflower rice for a low•carb meal.
• Top with your favorite marinara sauce and a sprinkle of parmesan cheese.
• Use the meatballs as a protein•rich snack or appetizer.
• Freeze any leftover meatballs for easy reheating later.

These baked Italian meatballs are a great option for an endomorph diet. The combination of ground beef and Italian sausage provides ample protein, while the almond flour and parmesan keep the carbs low. Adjust the portion sizes as needed to fit your individual macros.

51. Hard•boiled eggs

Ingredient:

• Large eggs

Instructions:

1. Place the eggs in a single layer in a saucepan and cover with cold water by 1 inch.

2. Bring the water to a boil over high heat.

3. Once the water reaches a rolling boil, remove the pan from the heat and cover with a lid.

4. Let the eggs sit in the hot water for the following times, depending on your desired doneness:
   • Soft•boiled: 6•7 minutes
   • Hard•boiled: 12 minutes

5. Drain the hot water and cover the eggs with cold water to stop the cooking process.

6. Let the eggs sit in the cold water for 5 minutes.

7. Peel the eggs and enjoy!

Tips:
• Older eggs peel more easily than very fresh eggs.
• To make peeling easier, add a teaspoon of baking soda to the cooking water.
• Store hard•boiled eggs in the refrigerator for up to 1 week.

Hard•boiled eggs are a fantastic option for an endomorph diet. They are high in protein, low in carbs, and can be easily incorporated into meals or enjoyed as a snack. The protein and healthy fats from the eggs will help keep you feeling full and satisfied. Adjust the portion size as needed to fit your individual macros.

52. Cucumber slices with hummus

Ingredient:

• 1 medium cucumber, sliced into rounds or sticks
• 1/2 cup hummus (store•bought or homemade)

Instructions:

1. Wash the cucumber and slice it into rounds or cut it into sticks, depending on your preference.

2. Scoop a small amount of hummus (about 1•2 tablespoons) onto each cucumber slice or stick.

3. Arrange the cucumber slices with hummus on a plate or in a container.

Optional Variations:
• Use different flavors of hummus, such as roasted red pepper, garlic, or Mediterranean.
• Top the hummus•topped cucumber slices with a sprinkle of:
  • Chopped fresh herbs (parsley, dill, or cilantro)
  • Crumbled feta cheese
  • Toasted sesame seeds
  • Paprika or cayenne pepper

This snack is a great option for an endomorph diet because:

• Cucumbers are low in calories and carbs, providing fiber and hydration.

• Hummus is a good source of plant•based protein and healthy fats from the tahini and olive oil.

• The combination of the crunchy cucumber and creamy hummus provides a satisfying and nutrient•dense snack.

Adjust the portion sizes as needed to fit your individual macros and calorie requirements. This makes for a simple, easy•to•prepare, and portable snack option.

53. Celery with almond butter

Ingredient:

- 2•3 stalks of celery, cut into 3•4 inch sticks
- 2•3 tablespoons of unsweetened almond butter

Instructions:

1. Wash the celery stalks and cut them into 3•4 inch sticks.

2. Scoop a small amount of almond butter (about 1•2 tablespoons) onto the end of each celery stick.

Optional Variations:

- Use different nut butters, such as peanut butter or cashew butter.

- Sprinkle a few chopped nuts or seeds on top of the almond butter for added crunch and texture.

- Drizzle a small amount of honey or maple syrup over the almond butter (in moderation for an endomorph diet).

- Dip the celery sticks in the almond butter instead of spreading it on top.

This snack is a great option for an endomorph diet because:

- Celery is low in calories and carbs, providing fiber and hydration.

- Almond butter is a good source of healthy fats and protein, which can help keep you feeling full and satisfied.

- The combination of the crunchy celery and creamy almond butter provides a satisfying and nutrient•dense snack.

Adjust the portion sizes as needed to fit your individual macros and calorie requirements. This makes for a simple, easy•to•prepare, and portable snack option.

54. Turkey roll•ups with avocado

Ingredient:

• 8 slices of deli turkey (about 4 oz)
• 1 ripe avocado, sliced
• 2 tbsp cream cheese, softened
• 1 tbsp chopped fresh cilantro (optional)
• Salt and pepper to taste

Instructions:

1. Lay the turkey slices out flat on a clean surface.

2. Spread about 1 tsp of the softened cream cheese evenly over each turkey slice.

3. Place a few slices of avocado in the center of each turkey slice.

4. Sprinkle the chopped cilantro (if using) over the avocado.

5. Season with a pinch of salt and pepper.

6. Carefully roll up each turkey slice, enclosing the avocado and cream cheese inside.

7. Secure the roll•ups with toothpicks, if needed.

8. Serve immediately or refrigerate until ready to enjoy.

Optional Variations:
• Use different types of deli meat, such as roast beef or ham.
• Add a thin slice of cheese, such as cheddar or provolone.
• Substitute the cream cheese with hummus or guacamole.
• Sprinkle the roll•ups with a dash of paprika or chili powder.

These turkey roll•ups with avocado are a great snack option for an endomorph diet. The turkey provides lean protein, the avocado offers healthy fats, and the cream cheese adds a creamy texture. Adjust the portion sizes as needed to fit your individual macros and calorie requirements.

55. Caprese skewers

Ingredient:

- 12 cherry or grape tomatoes
- 12 small fresh mozzarella balls (or cubes)
- 12 fresh basil leaves
- 2 tbsp balsamic glaze (or reduced•balsamic vinegar)
- 1 tbsp olive oil
- Salt and pepper to taste

Instructions:

1. Assemble the skewers by alternating a tomato, a mozzarella ball, and a basil leaf on each skewer.

2. Arrange the Caprese skewers on a serving platter.

3. Drizzle the balsamic glaze and olive oil over the skewers.

4. Season with a pinch of salt and pepper.

Optional Variations:
- Use different types of tomatoes, such as heirloom or sun•dried.
- Substitute the mozzarella with cubes of feta cheese.
- Add a small cube of avocado to each skewer.
- Sprinkle the skewers with a bit of grated Parmesan cheese.
- Serve the skewers with a side of balsamic vinegar for dipping.

These Caprese skewers are a great low•carb option for an endomorph diet. The tomatoes, mozzarella, and basil provide a classic flavor combination, while the balsamic glaze and olive oil add healthy fats. Adjust the portion sizes as needed to fit your individual macros and calorie requirements.

These skewers make for a simple, elegant, and portable snack or appetizer that's perfect for gatherings or as a healthy on•the•go option.

56. Roasted chickpeas

Ingredient:

• 1 (15 oz) can chickpeas (garbanzo beans), drained and rinsed
• 1 tbsp olive oil
• 1 tsp ground cumin
• 1 tsp paprika
• 1/2 tsp garlic powder
• 1/4 tsp cayenne pepper (optional)
• 1/4 tsp salt

Instructions:

1. Preheat your oven to 400°F. Line a baking sheet with parchment paper.

2. Pat the drained and rinsed chickpeas dry with a paper towel or clean kitchen towel.

3. In a medium bowl, toss the chickpeas with the olive oil, cumin, paprika, garlic powder, cayenne (if using), and salt until evenly coated.

4. Spread the seasoned chickpeas in a single layer on the prepared baking sheet.

5. Roast the chickpeas for 20•25 minutes, shaking the pan halfway, until they are crispy and golden brown.

6. Remove the roasted chickpeas from the oven and let them cool for 5 minutes before serving.

Flavor Variations:
• For a sweet and spicy version, add 1 tsp of honey or maple syrup to the seasoning mix.
• Try different spice blends, such as chili lime, ranch, or Italian seasoning.
• Toss the roasted chickpeas with grated parmesan cheese or chopped fresh herbs.

Roasted chickpeas make a great high•protein, low•carb snack for an endomorph diet. The fiber and protein from the chickpeas will help keep you feeling full and satisfied. Adjust the portion sizes as needed to fit your individual macros and calorie requirements.

These crunchy roasted chickpeas are also a versatile topping for salads, soups, or as a snack on their own.

57. Kale chips

Ingredient:

• 1 bunch of kale, washed and dried thoroughly
• 1•2 tbsp olive oil or avocado oil
• 1/2 tsp sea salt

Instructions:

1. Preheat your oven to 325°F (165°C).

2. Wash the kale and pat it completely dry with paper towels or a clean kitchen towel. Make sure there is no moisture left on the leaves, as this can prevent them from crisping up.

3. Tear the kale leaves into bite•sized pieces, discarding any tough stems.

4. Place the kale pieces in a large bowl and drizzle with the oil. Use your hands to massage the oil evenly over the kale.

5. Sprinkle the sea salt over the kale and toss to coat.

6. Arrange the kale pieces in a single layer on baking sheets lined with parchment paper or a silicone baking mat.

7. Bake for 12•15 minutes, flipping the kale halfway through, until the chips are crispy and lightly browned.

8. Remove from the oven and let cool completely before serving.

Kale is a nutrient•dense, low•calorie vegetable that can be a great addition to an endomorph diet. The healthy fats from the olive or avocado oil, along with the fiber and vitamins in the kale, make these chips a satisfying and nutritious snack.

58. Tuna salad cucumber boats

Ingredient:

- 2 (5 oz) cans of tuna, drained
- 2 tbsp plain Greek yogurt
- 1 tbsp Dijon mustard
- 1 tbsp lemon juice
- 2 tbsp finely chopped celery
- 2 tbsp finely chopped red onion
- 1 tbsp chopped fresh parsley
- Salt and pepper to taste
- 2 medium•sized cucumbers, halved lengthwise and scooped out to create "boats"

Instructions:

1. In a medium bowl, combine the drained tuna, Greek yogurt, Dijon mustard, lemon juice, celery, red onion, and parsley. Mix well until everything is evenly incorporated.

2. Season the tuna salad with salt and pepper to taste.

3. Scoop the tuna salad mixture into the hollowed•out cucumber boats, dividing it evenly among the 4 halves.

4. Serve the tuna salad cucumber boats chilled or at room temperature.

This recipe is a great option for an endomorph diet because it's high in protein from the tuna, low in carbs from the cucumber, and contains healthy fats from the yogurt and tuna. The vegetables also provide fiber and nutrients. It's a refreshing and satisfying snack or light meal.

59. Guacamole with veggie sticks

Ingredient:

- 3 ripe avocados, pitted and mashed
- 1/4 cup diced red onion
- 1 jalapeño, seeded and finely chopped (optional, for spice)
- 2 tbsp fresh lime juice
- 2 tbsp chopped fresh cilantro
- 1/2 tsp sea salt
- Assorted raw veggie sticks (such as carrot, celery, cucumber, bell pepper)

Instructions:

1. In a medium bowl, mash the avocados with a fork or potato masher until they reach your desired consistency (chunky or smooth).

2. Add the diced red onion, chopped jalapeño (if using), lime juice, chopped cilantro, and sea salt. Stir everything together until well combined.

3. Taste the guacamole and adjust any seasonings as needed, adding more lime juice for acidity, salt for flavor, or jalapeño for spice.

4. Arrange the assorted raw veggie sticks around the bowl of guacamole.

5. Serve the guacamole immediately with the veggie sticks for dipping.

This guacamole recipe is a great option for an endomorph diet because it's high in healthy fats from the avocado, low in carbs, and provides fiber and nutrients from the vegetables. The combination of the creamy guacamole and the crunchy veggie sticks makes for a satisfying and nutritious snack.

60. Smoked salmon cucumber rounds

Ingredient:

- 1 large cucumber, sliced into 1/4•inch thick rounds
- 4 oz smoked salmon, thinly sliced
- 2 tbsp cream cheese, softened
- 1 tbsp chopped fresh dill
- 1 tsp lemon juice
- Salt and pepper to taste

Instructions:

1. Slice the cucumber into 1/4•inch thick rounds and arrange them on a serving platter or plate.

2. In a small bowl, mix together the softened cream cheese, chopped dill, and lemon juice until well combined.

3. Top each cucumber round with a small dollop of the cream cheese mixture, spreading it to the edges.

4. Fold or roll up a small piece of smoked salmon and place it on top of the cream cheese on each cucumber round.

5. Season the tops of the smoked salmon cucumber rounds with a pinch of salt and pepper.

6. Serve chilled or at room temperature.

This recipe is a great option for an endomorph diet because it's low in carbs, high in healthy fats from the salmon and cream cheese, and provides a good source of protein. The cucumber rounds also add fiber and hydration. These smoked salmon cucumber rounds make for a refreshing and satisfying snack or appetizer.

61. Pumpkin seeds

Ingredient:

- 1 cup raw pumpkin seeds (pepitas)
- 1 tsp olive oil
- 1/2 tsp sea salt

Instructions:

1. Preheat your oven to 325°F (165°C).

2. Spread the raw pumpkin seeds out in a single layer on a baking sheet.

3. Drizzle the olive oil over the seeds and use your hands to toss and coat them evenly.

4. Sprinkle the sea salt over the seeds.

5. Roast the seeds for 15•20 minutes, stirring halfway, until lightly golden brown.

6. Allow the roasted pumpkin seeds to cool completely before serving.

Pumpkin seeds are a great snack for endomorphs as they are high in protein, fiber, and healthy fats, which can help keep you feeling full and satisfied. The roasting process also helps to enhance their nutty, savory flavor. Enjoy these as a nutritious snack or add them to salads, yogurt, or other dishes.

62. Edamame

Ingredient:

- 1 lb fresh edamame in the pod
- 1 tsp sea salt

Instructions:

1. Bring a large pot of water to a boil.

2. Add the edamame pods to the boiling water and cook for 5•7 minutes, until the pods are bright green and tender.

3. Drain the edamame and transfer to a serving bowl.

4. Sprinkle the sea salt over the hot edamame pods.

5. Serve the edamame warm, allowing guests to pop the beans out of the pods and enjoy.

Edamame is an excellent snack for endomorphs as it is high in protein, fiber, and complex carbohydrates, which can help keep blood sugar levels stable. The fiber and protein also help promote feelings of fullness.

This simple steamed preparation allows the natural flavors of the edamame to shine through. You can also experiment with other light seasonings like lemon juice, garlic powder, or a dash of soy sauce.

Enjoy this nutritious and satisfying snack as part of your endomorph diet plan.

63. Apple slices with peanut butter

Ingredient:

• 1 medium apple, cored and sliced
• 2 tbsp natural peanut butter (no added sugar or oils)

Instructions:

1. Wash and slice the apple into thin, even slices.

2. Spread about 1/2 to 1 tsp of peanut butter onto each apple slice.

That's it! This simple snack is a perfect combination of complex carbohydrates, healthy fats, and protein to keep you feeling full and satisfied.

The apple provides fiber, vitamins, and natural sweetness, while the peanut butter adds creaminess and a boost of plant•based protein and healthy monounsaturated fats. This is an ideal snack for endomorphs as it helps stabilize blood sugar levels and provides sustained energy.

You can use any type of apple you prefer, such as Gala, Fuji, or Honeycrisp. For the peanut butter, look for a natural variety with no added sugars or hydrogenated oils.

This snack is portable, easy to prepare, and can be enjoyed anytime as part of a balanced endomorph diet plan.

64. Turkey jerky

Ingredient:

- 1 lb boneless, skinless turkey breast, thinly sliced
- 2 tbsp Worcestershire sauce
- 1 tbsp soy sauce
- 1 tsp garlic powder
- 1 tsp onion powder
- 1 tsp black pepper
- 1/2 tsp smoked paprika (optional)
- 1/4 tsp red pepper flakes (optional)

Instructions:

1. In a large bowl, combine the Worcestershire sauce, soy sauce, garlic powder, onion powder, black pepper, smoked paprika (if using), and red pepper flakes (if using). Add the turkey slices and toss to coat evenly.

2. Cover the bowl and refrigerate for 2•4 hours, allowing the turkey to marinate.

3. Preheat your oven to 175°F (80°C). Line 2•3 baking sheets with parchment paper.

4. Arrange the marinated turkey slices in a single layer on the prepared baking sheets, making sure they are not overlapping.

5. Bake for 4•6 hours, flipping the jerky halfway through, until the turkey is dried and leathery. The exact time may vary depending on the thickness of your slices.

6. Allow the jerky to cool completely before storing in an airtight container at room temperature for up to 1 week.

Turkey jerky is an excellent high•protein, low•carb snack for endomorphs. It's portable, shelf•stable, and satisfying. The marinade adds great flavor without adding too many calories or carbs. Enjoy this homemade jerky as a healthy, energizing snack.

65. Cottage cheese with berries

Ingredient:

• 1 cup low•fat or non•fat cottage cheese
• 1/2 cup fresh or frozen berries (such as blueberries, raspberries, or blackberries)
• 1 tsp honey (optional)

Instructions:

1. Scoop the cottage cheese into a bowl.

2. Top the cottage cheese with the fresh or frozen berries.

3. If desired, drizzle the honey over the top.

That's it! This simple snack takes just a minute to prepare.

The cottage cheese provides a good amount of protein to help keep you feeling full, while the berries add natural sweetness, fiber, and antioxidants. The honey is optional, but can provide a touch of extra sweetness if desired.

This snack is perfect for endomorphs as it combines protein, complex carbs, and healthy fats to help stabilize blood sugar levels and provide sustained energy. The fiber from the berries also helps promote feelings of fullness.

You can use any type of berries you prefer, fresh or frozen. Feel free to experiment with different flavor combinations as well, such as adding a sprinkle of cinnamon or a few chopped nuts.

Enjoy this nutritious and satisfying cottage cheese and berry snack as part of your endomorph diet plan.

66. Nuts • almonds, walnuts, pistachios, etc.

Ingredient:

- 4 boneless, skinless chicken breasts
- 1 cup sliced almonds, finely chopped
- 1/2 cup grated Parmesan cheese
- 1 tsp dried oregano
- 1 tsp garlic powder
- 1/2 tsp salt
- 1/4 tsp black pepper
- 2 tbsp olive oil

Instructions:

1. Preheat oven to 400°F. Line a baking sheet with parchment paper.

2. In a shallow bowl, mix together the chopped almonds, Parmesan, oregano, garlic powder, salt, and pepper.

3. Brush the chicken breasts lightly with olive oil on both sides.

4. Dredge the chicken in the almond•Parmesan mixture, pressing it onto the chicken to help it adhere.

5. Place the coated chicken on the prepared baking sheet.

6. Bake for 25•30 minutes, until the chicken is cooked through and the coating is golden brown.

This dish is high in protein from the chicken and healthy fats from the almonds, making it a great option for an endomorph diet. The almond and Parmesan crust adds flavor and crunch without the need for breading or frying. Serve with a side of roasted vegetables for a complete, nutrient•dense meal.

67. String cheese

Ingredient:

- 1 gallon whole milk
- 1/4 cup white vinegar or lemon juice
- 1 tsp salt

Instructions:

1. In a large pot, bring the milk to a gentle simmer over medium heat, stirring occasionally to prevent scorching. Heat the milk to 185°F.

2. Once the milk reaches temperature, remove the pot from the heat and stir in the vinegar or lemon juice. The milk should start to curdle and separate into curds and whey.

3. Allow the mixture to sit for 5•10 minutes, until the curds have fully formed.

4. Drain the curds through a cheesecloth•lined colander, reserving the whey for another use if desired.

5. Gather the curds into a ball and knead them gently under cool running water until they become smooth and elastic, about 5•10 minutes.

6. Sprinkle the salt over the kneaded curds and continue kneading until the salt is fully incorporated.

7. Divide the cheese into 1•ounce portions and shape each into a string cheese stick.

8. Place the string cheese sticks in an airtight container in the refrigerator for up to 1 week.

This homemade string cheese is a great high•protein, low•carb snack for endomorphs. The whole milk provides healthy fats, while the minimal processing keeps the nutritional profile intact. Enjoy 1•2 sticks as a satisfying and portable snack.

68. Peanut butter protein balls

Ingredient:

- 1 cup natural peanut butter
- 1/2 cup rolled oats
- 1/4 cup vanilla protein powder
- 2 tbsp honey
- 1 tbsp chia seeds
- 1 tbsp ground flaxseed
- 1/4 tsp cinnamon

Instructions:

1. In a medium bowl, mix together the peanut butter, rolled oats, protein powder, honey, chia seeds, flaxseed, and cinnamon until well combined.

2. Scoop out tablespoon•sized portions of the mixture and roll them into balls with your hands.

3. Place the protein balls on a parchment•lined baking sheet and refrigerate for at least 30 minutes to allow them to firm up.

4. Store the protein balls in an airtight container in the refrigerator for up to 1 week.

These peanut butter protein balls are a great high•protein, high•fiber snack for endomorphs on a balanced diet. The peanut butter provides healthy fats, the oats and seeds offer complex carbs and fiber, and the protein powder helps support muscle growth and maintenance. Enjoy 1•2 balls as a nutritious pick•me•up!

69. Yogurt with low sugar granola

Ingredient:

- 1 cup plain Greek yogurt
- 1/2 cup low•sugar granola
- 1 tbsp chia seeds
- 1 tbsp sliced almonds
- 1 tsp honey (optional)

Instructions:

1. In a medium bowl, scoop out 1 cup of plain Greek yogurt.

2. Top the yogurt with 1/2 cup of low•sugar granola. Look for a granola that has less than 6•8 grams of sugar per serving.

3. Sprinkle 1 tablespoon of chia seeds and 1 tablespoon of sliced almonds over the granola.

4. If desired, drizzle 1 teaspoon of honey over the top for a touch of sweetness.

5. Stir everything together gently until well combined.

That's it! This simple yogurt and granola parfait makes for a nutritious and satisfying snack or light meal for endomorphs.

The Greek yogurt provides protein and probiotics, while the low•sugar granola offers complex carbs and fiber. The chia seeds and almonds add healthy fats, vitamins, and minerals. The optional honey provides a natural sweetener if needed.

This balanced combination of macronutrients and fiber will help keep you feeling full and energized between meals. Enjoy this yogurt parfait as a nutritious snack or breakfast.

70. Beef or turkey pepperoni slices

Ingredient:

- 1 lb ground beef or ground turkey
- 2 tsp smoked paprika
- 1 tsp garlic powder
- 1 tsp onion powder
- 1 tsp dried oregano
- 1 tsp fennel seeds (optional)
- 1 tsp red pepper flakes (optional)
- 1 tsp salt
- 1/2 tsp black pepper

Instructions:

1. In a large bowl, combine the ground beef or turkey with the smoked paprika, garlic powder, onion powder, dried oregano, fennel seeds (if using), red pepper flakes (if using), salt, and black pepper. Mix well until the spices are evenly distributed.

2. Line a baking sheet with parchment paper. Scoop the seasoned meat mixture onto the baking sheet and use your hands to shape it into a long, thin log about 1•inch thick.

3. Preheat your oven to 225°F. Bake the meat log for 2•3 hours, or until it is firm and cooked through. The internal temperature should reach 165°F.

4. Remove the baked meat log from the oven and let it cool completely. Once cooled, use a sharp knife to slice the log into thin, pepperoni•style slices.

5. Store the pepperoni slices in an airtight container in the refrigerator for up to 1 week.

These homemade beef or turkey pepperoni slices are a great high•protein, low•carb snack option for endomorphs. They can be enjoyed on their own, added to salads, or paired with cheese and vegetables. Adjust the spices to your desired level of heat and flavor.

71. Broccoli cheddar soup

Ingredient:

- 2 tbsp olive oil
- 1 onion, diced
- 3 cloves garlic, minced
- 4 cups low•sodium chicken or vegetable broth
- 4 cups chopped broccoli florets
- 1 cup shredded cheddar cheese
- 1/4 cup heavy cream (or unsweetened almond milk)
- 1 tsp Dijon mustard
- 1/2 tsp dried thyme
- Salt and pepper to taste

Instructions:

1. In a large pot, heat the olive oil over medium heat. Add the diced onion and sauté for 5 minutes until translucent.

2. Add the minced garlic and sauté for 1 minute until fragrant.

3. Pour in the broth and add the chopped broccoli florets. Bring the mixture to a boil, then reduce heat and simmer for 10•15 minutes until the broccoli is tender.

4. Using an immersion blender, carefully blend the soup until it reaches a creamy, smooth consistency. Alternatively, you can transfer the soup to a regular blender in batches.

5. Stir in the shredded cheddar cheese, heavy cream (or almond milk), Dijon mustard, and dried thyme. Season with salt and pepper to taste.

6. Simmer the soup for an additional 5 minutes, stirring occasionally, until the cheese is fully melted and the soup is heated through.

7. Serve hot, garnished with extra shredded cheddar cheese if desired.

This broccoli cheddar soup is a comforting and nutrient•dense option for endomorphs. The broccoli provides fiber and vitamins, while the cheddar cheese and cream add healthy fats to keep you feeling full and satisfied.

72. Chicken and vegetable soup

Ingredient:

• 1 lb boneless, skinless chicken breasts, cubed
• 1 tbsp olive oil
• 1 onion, diced
• 3 carrots, peeled and sliced
• 2 celery stalks, sliced
• 3 cloves garlic, minced
• 6 cups low•sodium chicken broth
• 2 cups chopped kale or spinach
• 1 tsp dried thyme
• 1 tsp dried oregano
• Salt and pepper to taste

Instructions:

1. In a large pot or Dutch oven, heat the olive oil over medium heat. Add the cubed chicken and cook for 3•4 minutes, until lightly browned.

2. Add the diced onion, sliced carrots, and sliced celery to the pot. Sauté for 5•7 minutes, until the vegetables start to soften.

3. Stir in the minced garlic and cook for 1 minute until fragrant.

4. Pour in the low•sodium chicken broth and add the chopped kale or spinach. Season with the dried thyme, dried oregano, salt, and pepper.

5. Bring the soup to a boil, then reduce the heat and let it simmer for 15•20 minutes, until the chicken is cooked through and the vegetables are tender.

6. Taste and adjust seasoning as needed. Serve the chicken and vegetable soup hot, garnished with extra chopped kale or parsley if desired.

This hearty and nutrient•dense soup is a great option for endomorphs on a balanced diet. The chicken provides lean protein, while the vegetables offer fiber, vitamins, and minerals. The broth•based soup is also hydrating and easy to digest.

Enjoy this soup as a satisfying main dish or a comforting side. It can be made in advance and stored in the refrigerator for up to 4 days.

73. Minestrone soup

Ingredient:

- 2 tbsp olive oil
- 1 onion, diced
- 3 cloves garlic, minced
- 2 carrots, peeled and diced
- 2 celery stalks, diced
- 1 zucchini, diced
- 1 tsp dried oregano
- 1 tsp dried basil
- Salt and pepper to taste
- 1 (15 oz) can diced tomatoes
- 4 cups low•sodium vegetable or chicken broth
- 1 (15 oz) can kidney beans, rinsed and drained
- 1 cup small whole wheat pasta (such as ditalini or elbow macaroni)
- 2 cups chopped kale or spinach

Instructions:

1. In a large pot or Dutch oven, heat the olive oil over medium heat. Add the diced onion and sauté for 5 minutes until translucent.

2. Add the minced garlic and sauté for 1 minute until fragrant.

3. Stir in the diced carrots, celery, and zucchini. Sauté for 5•7 minutes until the vegetables start to soften.

4. Pour in the can of diced tomatoes and the vegetable or chicken broth. Bring the mixture to a boil.

5. Once boiling, reduce the heat and let the soup simmer for 10 minutes.

6. Add the rinsed and drained kidney beans, the whole wheat pasta, and the chopped kale or spinach. Season with the dried oregano, dried basil, salt, and pepper.

7. Continue simmering the soup for an additional 10•15 minutes, until the pasta is tender and the greens are wilted.

8. Taste and adjust seasoning as needed. Serve the minestrone soup hot, garnished with extra chopped parsley or grated Parmesan cheese if desired.

This minestrone soup is a nutrient•dense and filling option for endomorphs. The combination of vegetables, beans, and whole grain pasta provides a balance of complex carbs, fiber, and protein to keep you satisfied.

74. Tomato basil soup

Ingredient:

• 2 tbsp olive oil
• 1 onion, diced
• 3 cloves garlic, minced
• 2 (28 oz) cans crushed tomatoes
• 2 cups low•sodium chicken or vegetable broth
• 1/4 cup fresh basil leaves, chopped
• 1 tsp dried oregano
• 1/4 tsp red pepper flakes (optional)
• 1/4 cup heavy cream or unsweetened almond milk
• Salt and pepper to taste

Instructions:

1. In a large pot or Dutch oven, heat the olive oil over medium heat. Add the diced onion and sauté for 5•7 minutes until translucent.

2. Add the minced garlic and sauté for 1 minute until fragrant.

3. Pour in the two cans of crushed tomatoes and the chicken or vegetable broth. Stir to combine.

4. Bring the soup to a simmer and let it cook for 10•15 minutes, stirring occasionally.

5. Remove the pot from the heat and stir in the chopped fresh basil, dried oregano, and red pepper flakes (if using).

6. Using an immersion blender, carefully blend the soup until it reaches a smooth, creamy consistency. Alternatively, you can transfer the soup to a regular blender in batches.

7. Stir in the heavy cream or unsweetened almond milk. Season with salt and pepper to taste.

8. Return the soup to low heat and let it simmer for an additional 5 minutes to allow the flavors to meld. Serve the tomato basil soup hot, garnished with extra fresh basil leaves if desired.

This tomato basil soup is a comforting and nutrient•dense option for endomorphs. The tomatoes provide lycopene and antioxidants, while the fresh basil and cream or almond milk add flavor and healthy fats. Enjoy this soup as a main dish or pair it with a side salad or whole grain crackers.

75. Egg drop soup

Ingredient:

- 4 cups low·sodium chicken broth
- 2 eggs, lightly beaten
- 2 tbsp low·sodium soy sauce
- 1 tsp sesame oil
- 1/2 tsp ground ginger
- 1/4 tsp white pepper
- 2 green onions, thinly sliced
- 1 cup shredded cooked chicken (optional)

Instructions:

1. In a medium saucepan, bring the low·sodium chicken broth to a gentle simmer over medium heat.

2. In a small bowl, lightly beat the 2 eggs.

3. Slowly drizzle the beaten eggs into the simmering broth in a circular motion, while gently stirring the broth with a fork or chopsticks. This will create delicate strands of cooked egg.

4. Once the egg has been incorporated, stir in the low·sodium soy sauce, sesame oil, ground ginger, and white pepper.

5. If using, add the shredded cooked chicken to the soup and stir to combine.

6. Remove the soup from heat and ladle into bowls. Top with the sliced green onions.

7. Serve the egg drop soup hot.

This egg drop soup is a light and nourishing option for endomorphs on a balanced diet. The protein·rich eggs and optional chicken provide satiety, while the broth and vegetables offer hydration and nutrients.

The minimal ingredients and simple preparation make this soup an easy and quick meal or snack. Adjust the seasoning to your taste preferences. Enjoy this egg drop soup on its own or with a side salad or whole grain crackers.

76. Beef and barley soup

Ingredient:

- 1 lb lean beef stew meat, cubed
- 2 tbsp olive oil
- 1 onion, diced
- 3 carrots, peeled and sliced
- 2 celery stalks, sliced
- 3 cloves garlic, minced
- 6 cups low•sodium beef or chicken broth
- 1 cup pearl barley
- 1 (14.5 oz) can diced tomatoes
- 2 tsp dried thyme
- 1 tsp dried rosemary
- Salt and pepper to taste

Instructions:

1. In a large pot or Dutch oven, heat the olive oil over medium•high heat. Add the cubed beef stew meat and brown on all sides, about 5•7 minutes total. Remove the beef from the pot and set aside.

2. Reduce the heat to medium and add the diced onion, sliced carrots, and sliced celery to the pot. Sauté for 5•7 minutes until the vegetables start to soften.

3. Stir in the minced garlic and cook for 1 minute until fragrant.

4. Pour in the low•sodium beef or chicken broth and add the pearl barley. Bring the mixture to a boil.

5. Once boiling, reduce the heat to low, return the browned beef to the pot, and add the can of diced tomatoes. Season with the dried thyme, dried rosemary, salt, and pepper.

6. Simmer the soup for 45•60 minutes, stirring occasionally, until the barley is tender and the beef is very tender.

7. Taste and adjust seasoning as needed. Serve the beef and barley soup hot, garnished with extra chopped parsley if desired.

This hearty and nutrient•dense soup is a great option for endomorphs on a balanced diet. The beef provides lean protein, while the barley offers complex carbs and fiber to help keep you feeling full and satisfied. The vegetables add vitamins, minerals, and antioxidants.

77. Butternut squash soup

Ingredient:

- 1 medium butternut squash, peeled, seeded, and cubed (about 4 cups)
- 1 tbsp olive oil
- 1 onion, diced
- 3 cloves garlic, minced
- 4 cups low•sodium chicken or vegetable broth
- 1/2 cup unsweetened almond milk
- 1 tsp ground cinnamon
- 1/2 tsp ground nutmeg
- Salt and pepper to taste
- Chopped parsley or pepitas for garnish (optional)

Instructions:

1. In a large pot or Dutch oven, heat the olive oil over medium heat. Add the diced onion and sauté for 5•7 minutes until translucent.

2. Add the minced garlic and sauté for 1 minute until fragrant.

3. Add the cubed butternut squash and the low•sodium broth to the pot. Bring the mixture to a boil.

4. Once boiling, reduce the heat to medium•low and let the soup simmer for 20•25 minutes, or until the squash is very soft.

5. Remove the pot from the heat and use an immersion blender to puree the soup until smooth and creamy. Alternatively, you can transfer the soup to a regular blender in batches.

6. Stir in the unsweetened almond milk, ground cinnamon, and ground nutmeg. Season with salt and pepper to taste.

7. Return the soup to low heat and let it simmer for an additional 5 minutes to allow the flavors to meld. Ladle the butternut squash soup into bowls and garnish with chopped parsley or pepitas, if desired.

This butternut squash soup is a comforting and nutrient•dense option for endomorphs. The squash provides complex carbs, fiber, and vitamins, while the almond milk adds healthy fats to help keep you feeling full and satisfied. Enjoy this soup as a main dish or pair it with a side salad or whole grain crackers.

78. Split pea and ham soup

Ingredient:

- 1 tbsp olive oil
- 1 onion, diced
- 3 carrots, peeled and diced
- 2 celery stalks, diced
- 3 cloves garlic, minced
- 1 lb dried split peas, rinsed
- 6 cups low•sodium chicken or vegetable broth
- 1 cup diced cooked ham
- 1 bay leaf
- 1 tsp dried thyme
- Salt and pepper to taste

Instructions:

1. In a large pot or Dutch oven, heat the olive oil over medium heat. Add the diced onion, carrots, and celery. Sauté for 5•7 minutes until the vegetables start to soften.

2. Stir in the minced garlic and cook for 1 minute until fragrant.

3. Add the rinsed dried split peas, low•sodium broth, diced cooked ham, bay leaf, and dried thyme. Bring the mixture to a boil.

4. Once boiling, reduce the heat to low, cover the pot, and let the soup simmer for 45•60 minutes, stirring occasionally, until the split peas are very soft and the soup has thickened.

5. Remove the bay leaf. Use an immersion blender to partially puree the soup, leaving some texture. Alternatively, you can transfer a portion of the soup to a regular blender and blend until smooth, then return it to the pot.

6. Season the split pea and ham soup with salt and pepper to taste. Serve the soup hot, garnished with extra chopped parsley or a drizzle of olive oil if desired.

This split pea and ham soup is a hearty and nutrient•dense option for endomorphs. The split peas provide complex carbs and fiber, while the ham adds lean protein. The vegetables contribute vitamins, minerals, and antioxidants.

This soup can be made in advance and stored in the refrigerator for up to 4 days. It also freezes well for longer•term storage.

79. Turkey chili

Ingredient:

- 1 lb ground turkey
- 1 tbsp olive oil
- 1 onion, diced
- 3 cloves garlic, minced
- 2 bell peppers, diced
- 2 (15 oz) cans diced tomatoes
- 1 (15 oz) can kidney beans, rinsed and drained
- 1 (15 oz) can black beans, rinsed and drained
- 2 tbsp chili powder
- 1 tsp ground cumin
- 1 tsp dried oregano
- 1/2 tsp smoked paprika
- 1/4 tsp cayenne pepper (optional)
- Salt and pepper to taste
- Chopped cilantro for garnish (optional)

Instructions:

1. In a large pot or Dutch oven, heat the olive oil over medium•high heat. Add the ground turkey and cook, breaking it up with a wooden spoon, until browned, about 5•7 minutes.

2. Add the diced onion, minced garlic, and diced bell peppers to the pot. Sauté for 5•7 minutes until the vegetables start to soften.

3. Stir in the two cans of diced tomatoes, the rinsed and drained kidney and black beans, chili powder, cumin, dried oregano, smoked paprika, and cayenne pepper (if using). Season with salt and pepper.

4. Bring the chili to a simmer, then reduce the heat to medium•low. Let the chili simmer for 20•30 minutes, stirring occasionally, until the flavors have melded and the chili has thickened.

5. Taste and adjust seasoning as needed. Serve the turkey chili hot, garnished with chopped cilantro if desired.

This turkey chili is a great option for endomorphs on a balanced diet. The ground turkey provides lean protein, while the beans offer complex carbs and fiber to help keep you feeling full and satisfied. The vegetables and spices add flavor, vitamins, and antioxidants.

80. Beef stew

Ingredient:

- 1 lb beef stew meat, cubed
- 2 tbsp olive oil
- 1 onion, diced
- 3 carrots, peeled and diced
- 2 celery stalks, diced
- 3 cloves garlic, minced
- 4 cups low•sodium beef broth
- 1 (14.5 oz) can diced tomatoes
- 2 bay leaves
- 1 tsp dried thyme
- 1 tsp dried rosemary
- 2 medium potatoes, peeled and cubed
- Salt and pepper to taste
- Chopped parsley for garnish (optional)

Instructions:

1. In a large pot or Dutch oven, heat the olive oil over medium•high heat. Add the cubed beef stew meat and brown on all sides, about 5•7 minutes total. Remove the beef from the pot and set aside.

2. Reduce the heat to medium and add the diced onion, carrots, and celery to the pot. Sauté for 5•7 minutes until the vegetables start to soften.

3. Stir in the minced garlic and cook for 1 minute until fragrant.

4. Pour in the low•sodium beef broth and add the can of diced tomatoes, bay leaves, dried thyme, and dried rosemary. Season with salt and pepper.

5. Return the browned beef to the pot and bring the stew to a boil.

6. Once boiling, reduce the heat to low, cover the pot, and let the stew simmer for 45•60 minutes, stirring occasionally.

7. Add the peeled and cubed potatoes to the pot and continue simmering for an additional 20•30 minutes, until the beef and potatoes are very tender.

8. Remove the bay leaves. Taste and adjust seasoning as needed. Serve the beef stew hot, garnished with chopped parsley if desired.

This hearty beef stew is a comforting and nutrient•dense option for endomorphs. The beef provides lean protein, while the vegetables and potatoes offer complex carbs, fiber, and essential vitamins and minerals. The broth•based stew is also hydrating and easy to digest.

81. Clam chowder (without potatoes)

Ingredient:

- 2 tbsp olive oil
- 1 onion, diced
- 2 celery stalks, diced
- 2 carrots, peeled and diced
- 3 cloves garlic, minced
- 2 (6.5 oz) cans chopped clams, with juice
- 2 cups unsweetened almond milk
- 1 cup low•sodium chicken or vegetable broth
- 1 tsp dried thyme
- 1/2 tsp dried oregano
- 1/4 tsp cayenne pepper (optional)
- Salt and pepper to taste
- Chopped parsley for garnish (optional)

Instructions:

1. In a large pot or Dutch oven, heat the olive oil over medium heat. Add the diced onion, celery, and carrots. Sauté for 5•7 minutes until the vegetables start to soften.

2. Stir in the minced garlic and cook for 1 minute until fragrant.

3. Add the two cans of chopped clams, including the juice, to the pot. Pour in the unsweetened almond milk and low•sodium broth.

4. Season the chowder with the dried thyme, dried oregano, cayenne pepper (if using), salt, and pepper.

5. Bring the chowder to a simmer and let it cook for 15•20 minutes, stirring occasionally, until the vegetables are tender.

6. Taste and adjust seasoning as needed. Serve the clam chowder hot, garnished with chopped parsley if desired.

This clam chowder recipe omits the traditional potatoes to keep it lower in carbs and more suitable for an endomorph diet. The almond milk provides a creamy texture without the need for heavy cream or potatoes.

The clams offer a good source of protein, while the vegetables contribute fiber, vitamins, and minerals. This chowder can be enjoyed as a main dish or as a side to a larger meal.

82. Chicken tortilla•less soup

Ingredient:

- 1 lb boneless, skinless chicken breasts, cubed
- 2 tbsp olive oil
- 1 onion, diced
- 3 cloves garlic, minced
- 2 bell peppers, diced
- 4 cups low•sodium chicken broth
- 1 (14.5 oz) can diced tomatoes
- 1 tsp ground cumin
- 1 tsp chili powder
- 1/2 tsp dried oregano
- Salt and pepper to taste
- Toppings (optional): avocado, shredded cheese, chopped cilantro, lime wedges

Instructions:

1. In a large pot or Dutch oven, heat the olive oil over medium•high heat. Add the cubed chicken and cook, stirring occasionally, until browned on all sides, about 5•7 minutes.

2. Reduce the heat to medium and add the diced onion, minced garlic, and diced bell peppers to the pot. Sauté for 5•7 minutes until the vegetables start to soften.

3. Pour in the low•sodium chicken broth and the can of diced tomatoes. Season with the ground cumin, chili powder, dried oregano, salt, and pepper.

4. Bring the soup to a simmer and let it cook for 15•20 minutes, until the chicken is cooked through and the vegetables are tender.

5. Taste and adjust seasoning as needed.

6. Serve the chicken tortilla•less soup hot, allowing guests to top their bowls with desired toppings such as avocado, shredded cheese, chopped cilantro, and lime wedges.

This chicken tortilla•less soup is a delicious and nutrient•dense option for endomorphs. The chicken provides lean protein, while the vegetables offer fiber, vitamins, and minerals. By omitting the traditional tortilla strips, you keep the carb content lower and more suitable for an endomorph diet.

Feel free to adjust the spices to your taste preferences. This soup can be made in advance and stored in the refrigerator for up to 4 days.

83. Italian wedding soup

Ingredient:

- 1 lb ground turkey or lean ground beef
- 1/4 cup grated Parmesan cheese
- 2 tbsp almond flour
- 1 egg, lightly beaten
- 2 tsp dried parsley
- 1 tsp garlic powder
- Salt and pepper to taste
- 2 tbsp olive oil
- 1 onion, diced
- 3 carrots, peeled and sliced
- 2 celery stalks, sliced
- 4 cups low•sodium chicken broth
- 2 cups chopped kale or spinach
- 1/2 cup small whole wheat pasta
(such as ditalini or acini de pepe)

Instructions:

1. In a medium bowl, combine the ground turkey/beef, Parmesan cheese, almond flour, egg, dried parsley, garlic powder, salt, and pepper. Mix well and form into small meatballs, about 1•inch in size.

2. In a large pot or Dutch oven, heat the olive oil over medium heat. Add the diced onion, sliced carrots, and sliced celery. Sauté for 5•7 minutes until the vegetables start to soften.

3. Pour in the low•sodium chicken broth and bring the mixture to a simmer.

4. Carefully add the meatballs and the whole wheat pasta to the simmering broth. Cook for 10•12 minutes, until the meatballs are cooked through and the pasta is tender.

5. Stir in the chopped kale or spinach and cook for an additional 2•3 minutes, until the greens are wilted.

6. Taste and adjust seasoning as needed. Serve the Italian wedding soup hot, garnished with extra grated Parmesan cheese if desired.

This Italian wedding soup is a hearty and nutrient•dense option for endomorphs. The lean turkey or beef meatballs provide protein, while the vegetables, broth, and whole grain pasta offer complex carbs, fiber, and essential vitamins and minerals.

The almond flour helps bind the meatballs without adding too many carbs. This soup can be made in advance and stored in the refrigerator for up to 4 days.

84. French onion soup

Ingredient:

- 3 tbsp olive oil
- 4 large onions, thinly sliced
- 2 cloves garlic, minced
- 1/4 cup dry white wine (or low•sodium beef broth)
- 4 cups low•sodium beef broth
- 1 tsp dried thyme
- 1/2 tsp dried rosemary
- Salt and pepper to taste
- 1/2 cup shredded low•fat mozzarella or provolone cheese

Instructions:

1. In a large pot or Dutch oven, heat the olive oil over medium heat. Add the thinly sliced onions and sauté for 20•25 minutes, stirring occasionally, until the onions are very soft and caramelized.

2. Stir in the minced garlic and cook for 1 minute until fragrant.

3. Deglaze the pot by pouring in the dry white wine (or low•sodium beef broth) and scraping up any browned bits from the bottom of the pot.

4. Add the low•sodium beef broth, dried thyme, and dried rosemary. Season with salt and pepper.

5. Bring the soup to a simmer and let it cook for 15•20 minutes, allowing the flavors to meld.

6. Preheat your oven's broiler.

7. Ladle the French onion soup into oven•safe bowls or ramekins. Top each serving with a couple tablespoons of the shredded low•fat mozzarella or provolone cheese.

8. Place the bowls on a baking sheet and broil for 2•3 minutes, or until the cheese is melted and bubbly. Serve the French onion soup hot, garnished with extra chopped parsley if desired.

This French onion soup is a comforting and flavorful option for endomorphs. The caramelized onions provide natural sweetness, while the low•fat cheese adds a touch of creaminess without too many calories or carbs.

85. Mushroom soup

Ingredient:

- 2 tbsp olive oil
- 1 lb mixed mushrooms (such as cremini, shiitake, and oyster), sliced
- 1 onion, diced
- 3 cloves garlic, minced
- 4 cups low·sodium chicken or vegetable broth
- 1/2 cup unsweetened almond milk
- 2 tbsp almond flour
- 1 tsp dried thyme
- Salt and pepper to taste
- Chopped parsley for garnish (optional)

Instructions:

1. In a large pot or Dutch oven, heat the olive oil over medium·high heat. Add the sliced mushrooms and sauté for 5·7 minutes, until they start to brown.

2. Reduce the heat to medium and add the diced onion to the pot. Sauté for 5·7 minutes until the onion is translucent.

3. Stir in the minced garlic and cook for 1 minute until fragrant.

4. Pour in the low·sodium broth and bring the mixture to a simmer.

5. In a small bowl, whisk together the unsweetened almond milk and almond flour until smooth. Slowly pour this mixture into the simmering soup, whisking constantly, to thicken the soup.

6. Stir in the dried thyme and season with salt and pepper to taste.

7. Reduce the heat to low and let the soup simmer for 10·15 minutes, stirring occasionally, until it has reached your desired consistency. Ladle the creamy mushroom soup into bowls and garnish with chopped parsley if desired.

This mushroom soup is a rich and satisfying option for endomorphs. The mushrooms provide umami flavor, while the almond milk and flour create a creamy texture without the need for heavy cream. The broth·based soup is also hydrating and easy to digest.

Enjoy this soup as a main course or pair it with a side salad or roasted vegetables for a complete meal.

86. Cobb salad

Ingredient:

- 6 cups chopped romaine lettuce
- 1 cup chopped cooked chicken breast
- 2 hard·boiled eggs, chopped
- 1/2 cup diced avocado
- 1/2 cup diced tomatoes
- 2 slices cooked turkey bacon, crumbled
- 2 tbsp crumbled feta cheese
- 2 tbsp olive oil
- 1 tbsp red wine vinegar
- 1 tsp Dijon mustard
- 1 tsp honey
- Salt and pepper to taste

Instructions:

1. In a large salad bowl, arrange the chopped romaine lettuce.

2. Top the lettuce with the cooked chicken breast, chopped hard·boiled eggs, diced avocado, diced tomatoes, crumbled turkey bacon, and crumbled feta cheese.

3. In a small bowl, whisk together the olive oil, red wine vinegar, Dijon mustard, and honey to make the dressing. Season with salt and pepper.

4. Drizzle the dressing over the salad and toss gently to coat.

5. Serve the Cobb salad immediately.

This Cobb salad is a nutrient·dense and filling option for endomorphs. The romaine lettuce, tomatoes, and avocado provide fiber, vitamins, and healthy fats. The chicken and eggs offer lean protein, while the turkey bacon and feta cheese add flavor and a touch of richness.

The simple vinaigrette dressing ties all the flavors together without adding too many extra calories or carbs.

Feel free to adjust the ingredient amounts to your taste preferences. This Cobb salad makes for a satisfying main dish or can be served as a side salad.

87. Spinach salad with bacon and eggs

Ingredient:

- 6 cups baby spinach leaves
- 4 hard•boiled eggs, sliced
- 4 slices turkey bacon, cooked and crumbled
- 1/4 cup sliced mushrooms
- 2 tbsp diced red onion
- 2 tbsp olive oil
- 1 tbsp red wine vinegar
- 1 tsp Dijon mustard
- 1 tsp honey
- Salt and pepper to taste

Instructions:

1. In a large salad bowl, combine the baby spinach leaves, sliced hard•boiled eggs, crumbled turkey bacon, sliced mushrooms, and diced red onion.

2. In a small bowl, whisk together the olive oil, red wine vinegar, Dijon mustard, and honey to make the dressing. Season with salt and pepper.

3. Drizzle the dressing over the salad and toss gently to coat.

4. Serve the spinach salad immediately.

This spinach salad is a nutrient•dense and satisfying option for endomorphs. The spinach provides fiber, vitamins, and antioxidants. The hard•boiled eggs and turkey bacon offer lean protein to help keep you feeling full.

The healthy fats from the olive oil and avocado in the dressing help slow the absorption of the carbs from the spinach, preventing blood sugar spikes.

Feel free to adjust the ingredient amounts to your taste preferences. You can also add other toppings like sliced avocado, shredded cheese, or toasted nuts if desired.

This spinach salad makes for a great main dish or can be served as a side salad.

88. Greek salad

Ingredient:

- 6 cups chopped romaine lettuce
- 1 cup diced cucumber
- 1/2 cup diced tomatoes
- 1/4 cup diced red onion
- 1/4 cup pitted kalamata olives, halved
- 2 oz crumbled feta cheese
- 2 tbsp olive oil
- 1 tbsp red wine vinegar
- 1 tsp dried oregano
- 1/2 tsp Dijon mustard
- Salt and pepper to taste

Instructions:

1. In a large salad bowl, combine the chopped romaine lettuce, diced cucumber, diced tomatoes, diced red onion, and halved kalamata olives.

2. Sprinkle the crumbled feta cheese over the top of the salad.

3. In a small bowl, whisk together the olive oil, red wine vinegar, dried oregano, and Dijon mustard to make the dressing. Season with salt and pepper.

4. Drizzle the dressing over the salad and toss gently to coat.

5. Serve the Greek salad immediately.

This Greek salad is a refreshing and nutrient•dense option for endomorphs. The romaine lettuce, cucumber, and tomatoes provide fiber, vitamins, and antioxidants. The feta cheese and olives add healthy fats and bold flavor.

The simple vinaigrette dressing ties all the flavors together without adding too many extra calories or carbs.

You can customize this salad by adding grilled chicken or shrimp for extra protein, or by substituting different vegetables based on your preferences.

This Greek salad makes for a great main dish or can be served as a side to a larger meal.

89. Broccoli salad

Ingredient:

- 4 cups broccoli florets, chopped
- 1/2 cup diced red onion
- 1/2 cup shredded cheddar cheese
- 3 slices cooked turkey bacon, crumbled
- 1/4 cup unsweetened dried cranberries
- 2 tbsp olive oil
- 2 tbsp apple cider vinegar
- 1 tsp Dijon mustard
- 1 tsp honey
- Salt and pepper to taste

Instructions:

1. In a large bowl, combine the chopped broccoli florets, diced red onion, shredded cheddar cheese, crumbled turkey bacon, and unsweetened dried cranberries.

2. In a small bowl, whisk together the olive oil, apple cider vinegar, Dijon mustard, and honey to make the dressing. Season with salt and pepper.

3. Pour the dressing over the broccoli salad and toss gently to coat.

4. Cover the salad and refrigerate for at least 30 minutes to allow the flavors to meld.

5. Serve the broccoli salad chilled or at room temperature.

This broccoli salad is a nutrient•dense and flavorful option for endomorphs. The broccoli provides fiber, vitamins, and antioxidants. The cheddar cheese and turkey bacon add protein and healthy fats to help keep you feeling full.

The dried cranberries provide a touch of natural sweetness, while the vinaigrette dressing ties all the flavors together.

You can customize this salad by adding other crunchy vegetables, such as shredded carrots or sliced almonds, or by substituting different types of cheese or protein.

This broccoli salad makes for a great side dish or can be enjoyed as a main course.

90. Kale Caesar salad

Ingredient:

- 6 cups chopped kale leaves
- 1/4 cup grated Parmesan cheese
- 2 tbsp olive oil
- 2 tbsp lemon juice
- 1 tbsp Dijon mustard
- 1 tsp Worcestershire sauce
- 1 clove garlic, minced
- Salt and pepper to taste
- 1/4 cup roasted unsalted almonds, chopped

Instructions:

1. In a large salad bowl, combine the chopped kale leaves and grated Parmesan cheese.

2. In a small bowl, whisk together the olive oil, lemon juice, Dijon mustard, Worcestershire sauce, and minced garlic to make the Caesar dressing. Season with salt and pepper.

3. Pour the Caesar dressing over the kale and Parmesan, and toss the salad until the leaves are evenly coated.

4. Sprinkle the chopped roasted almonds over the top of the salad.

5. Cover the salad and refrigerate for at least 15 minutes to allow the kale to soften and the flavors to meld. Serve the kale Caesar salad chilled or at room temperature.

This kale Caesar salad is a nutrient·dense and satisfying option for endomorphs. The kale provides fiber, vitamins, and antioxidants, while the Parmesan cheese and roasted almonds add protein and healthy fats.

The homemade Caesar dressing is made without heavy cream or egg yolks, keeping the calorie and carb content lower. The lemon juice and Dijon mustard help balance the flavors.

You can customize this salad by adding grilled chicken or shrimp for extra protein, or by substituting different types of nuts or seeds.

This kale Caesar salad makes for a great main dish or can be served as a side to a larger meal.

91. Salmon avocado salad

Ingredient:

- 4 cups mixed greens (such as spinach, arugula, and kale)
- 1 (6 oz) can wild•caught salmon, drained and flaked
- 1 avocado, diced
- 1/4 cup diced cucumber
- 2 tbsp sliced red onion
- 2 tbsp olive oil
- 1 tbsp apple cider vinegar
- 1 tsp Dijon mustard
- 1 tsp honey
- Salt and pepper to taste

Instructions:

1. In a large salad bowl, combine the mixed greens, flaked salmon, diced avocado, diced cucumber, and sliced red onion.

2. In a small bowl, whisk together the olive oil, apple cider vinegar, Dijon mustard, and honey to make the dressing. Season with salt and pepper.

3. Drizzle the dressing over the salad and toss gently to coat.

4. Serve the salmon avocado salad immediately.

This salmon avocado salad is a nutrient•dense and filling option for endomorphs. The salmon provides lean protein and healthy omega•3 fatty acids, while the avocado offers heart•healthy monounsaturated fats.

The mixed greens, cucumber, and red onion provide fiber, vitamins, and antioxidants to round out the salad. The simple vinaigrette dressing ties all the flavors together without adding too many extra calories or carbs.

You can customize this salad by adding other toppings like cherry tomatoes, sliced radishes, or toasted nuts and seeds. The salmon can also be substituted with grilled or baked chicken breast for a different protein option.

Enjoy this salmon avocado salad as a main dish or as a side to a larger meal.

92. Steak salad with blue cheese

Ingredient:

- 6 oz grilled or pan•seared steak, sliced
- 4 cups mixed greens (such as spinach, arugula, and romaine)
- 1/2 cup cherry tomatoes, halved
- 1/4 cup crumbled blue cheese
- 2 tbsp sliced red onion
- 2 tbsp olive oil
- 1 tbsp balsamic vinegar
- 1 tsp Dijon mustard
- 1 tsp honey
- Salt and pepper to taste

Instructions:

1. In a large salad bowl, combine the mixed greens, cherry tomatoes, crumbled blue cheese, and sliced red onion.

2. Top the salad with the sliced grilled or pan•seared steak.

3. In a small bowl, whisk together the olive oil, balsamic vinegar, Dijon mustard, and honey to make the dressing. Season with salt and pepper.

4. Drizzle the dressing over the steak salad and toss gently to coat.

5. Serve the steak salad with blue cheese immediately.

This steak salad is a satisfying and nutrient•dense option for endomorphs. The grilled or pan•seared steak provides lean protein, while the mixed greens, tomatoes, and onion offer fiber, vitamins, and antioxidants.

The crumbled blue cheese adds a creamy, tangy flavor and healthy fats to the salad. The balsamic vinaigrette dressing ties all the flavors together without adding too many extra calories or carbs.

You can customize this salad by adjusting the amount of steak, cheese, or vegetables based on your preferences. You can also add other toppings like avocado, roasted nuts, or hard•boiled eggs.

This steak salad makes for a great main dish or can be served as a side to a larger meal.

93. Caprese salad

Ingredient:

- 8 oz fresh mozzarella cheese, sliced
- 3 medium tomatoes, sliced
- 1/4 cup fresh basil leaves
- 2 tbsp extra virgin olive oil
- 1 tbsp balsamic vinegar
- Salt and pepper to taste

Instructions:

1. Arrange the sliced mozzarella and tomatoes on a serving platter or plate in an overlapping pattern.

2. Scatter the fresh basil leaves over the top.

3. Drizzle the olive oil and balsamic vinegar over the salad.

4. Season with salt and freshly ground black pepper to taste.

5. Let the salad sit for 5•10 minutes to allow the flavors to meld together.

6. Serve immediately.

Tips:
- Use the freshest, ripest tomatoes you can find for the best flavor.
- For extra flavor, you can add a sprinkle of dried oregano or a pinch of red pepper flakes.
- Serve with crusty bread or crackers on the side.

94. Asian chicken salad

Ingredient:

• 4 cups shredded cooked chicken breast
• 4 cups shredded cabbage (or coleslaw mix)
• 1 cup shredded carrots
• 1/2 cup sliced cucumber
• 1/4 cup sliced green onions
• 2 tbsp toasted sesame seeds
• 2 tbsp rice vinegar
• 1 tbsp sesame oil
• 1 tbsp low•sodium soy sauce
• 1 tsp honey
• 1 tsp Dijon mustard
• Salt and pepper to taste

Instructions:
1. In a large salad bowl, combine the shredded cooked chicken, shredded cabbage, shredded carrots, sliced cucumber, and sliced green onions.

2. In a small bowl, whisk together the rice vinegar, sesame oil, low•sodium soy sauce, honey, and Dijon mustard to make the dressing. Season with salt and pepper.

3. Pour the dressing over the salad and toss gently to coat.

4. Sprinkle the toasted sesame seeds over the top of the salad.

5. Serve the Asian chicken salad immediately.

This Asian chicken salad is a flavorful and nutrient•dense option for endomorphs. The shredded chicken provides lean protein, while the cabbage, carrots, and cucumber offer fiber, vitamins, and antioxidants.

The sesame oil and rice vinegar dressing adds a delicious Asian•inspired flavor profile without too many extra calories or carbs. The toasted sesame seeds provide a nice crunch.

You can customize this salad by adding other crunchy vegetables like bell peppers or snap peas, or by substituting the protein with grilled or baked tofu for a vegetarian option.

95. Taco salad (no shell)

Ingredient:

- 4 oz lean ground turkey or beef
- 1 tbsp taco seasoning
- 4 cups chopped romaine lettuce
- 1/2 cup diced tomatoes
- 1/4 cup diced red onion
- 1/4 cup sliced black olives
- 1/4 cup shredded cheddar cheese
- 2 tbsp plain Greek yogurt
- 1 tbsp fresh cilantro, chopped
- Juice of 1 lime
- Salt and pepper to taste

Instructions:

1. In a skillet over medium heat, cook the ground turkey/beef and taco seasoning until browned and cooked through, 5•7 minutes. Drain any excess fat.

2. In a large salad bowl, combine the chopped romaine, tomatoes, onion, olives, and shredded cheese.

3. Top the salad with the cooked seasoned ground meat.

4. In a small bowl, mix together the Greek yogurt, cilantro, and lime juice. Season with salt and pepper.

5. Drizzle the yogurt dressing over the salad and toss gently to coat.

Nutrition Info (per serving):
Calories: 300
Protein: 30g
Carbs: 15g
Fat: 15g
Fiber: 5g

This taco salad is a great option for an endomorph diet as it's high in protein, moderate in carbs, and low in fat. The Greek yogurt dressing provides a creamy texture without added calories or fat. Enjoy!

96. Shrimp avocado salad

Ingredient:

- 1 lb cooked shrimp, peeled and deveined
- 2 avocados, diced
- 1 cup cherry tomatoes, halved
- 1/2 cup diced red onion
- 1/4 cup chopped fresh cilantro
- 2 tbsp fresh lime juice
- 1 tbsp extra virgin olive oil
- 1 tsp Dijon mustard
- Salt and pepper to taste

Instructions:

1. In a large bowl, gently toss together the cooked shrimp, diced avocado, cherry tomatoes, red onion, and cilantro.

2. In a small bowl, whisk together the lime juice, olive oil, and Dijon mustard. Season with salt and pepper.

3. Drizzle the dressing over the shrimp and avocado salad and toss gently to coat.

4. Serve immediately or refrigerate until ready to serve.

Nutrition Info (per serving):
Calories: 280
Protein: 25g
Carbs: 12g
Fat: 16g
Fiber: 7g

This shrimp avocado salad is a great option for an endomorph diet. It's high in protein from the shrimp, healthy fats from the avocado, and low in carbs. The lime juice and Dijon dressing adds flavor without added sugar or calories. Enjoy this refreshing and nutritious salad!

97. Waldorf salad

Ingredient:

- 2 cups chopped romaine lettuce
- 1 cup diced apples (about 1 medium apple)
- 1/2 cup diced celery
- 1/4 cup chopped walnuts
- 2 tbsp plain Greek yogurt
- 1 tbsp lemon juice
- 1 tsp honey
- Salt and pepper to taste

Instructions:

1. In a large bowl, combine the chopped romaine lettuce, diced apples, celery, and walnuts.

2. In a small bowl, whisk together the Greek yogurt, lemon juice, and honey. Season with a pinch of salt and pepper.

3. Drizzle the yogurt dressing over the salad and toss gently to coat.

4. Serve immediately.

Nutrition Info (per serving):
Calories: 150
Protein: 7g
Carbs: 15g
Fat: 8g
Fiber: 4g

This Waldorf salad is a great option for an endomorph diet. It's lower in carbs and higher in protein and healthy fats compared to a traditional Waldorf salad. The Greek yogurt dressing provides creaminess without added sugar or calories. The apples, celery, and walnuts add crunch and fiber. Enjoy this refreshing and satisfying salad!

98. Cucumber tomato salad

Ingredient:

- 2 cups diced cucumber
- 1 cup halved cherry tomatoes
- 1/4 cup diced red onion
- 2 tbsp crumbled feta cheese
- 2 tbsp fresh chopped basil
- 1 tbsp red wine vinegar
- 1 tbsp extra virgin olive oil
- 1 tsp Dijon mustard
- Salt and pepper to taste

Instructions:

1. In a large bowl, combine the diced cucumber, halved cherry tomatoes, and diced red onion.

2. In a small bowl, whisk together the red wine vinegar, olive oil, and Dijon mustard. Season with a pinch of salt and pepper.

3. Drizzle the vinaigrette over the cucumber and tomato mixture and toss gently to coat.

4. Sprinkle the crumbled feta cheese and chopped fresh basil over the top.

5. Serve immediately or refrigerate until ready to serve.

Nutrition Info (per serving):
Calories: 100
Protein: 3g
Carbs: 8g
Fat: 7g
Fiber: 2g

This cucumber tomato salad is a great option for an endomorph diet. It's low in calories and carbs, but high in fiber, vitamins, and healthy fats from the olive oil and feta. The vinaigrette dressing adds flavor without added sugar. Enjoy this refreshing and nutritious salad!

99. Antipasto salad

Ingredient:

- 6 cups chopped romaine lettuce
- 1 cup halved cherry tomatoes
- 1/2 cup diced cucumber
- 1/2 cup diced red onion
- 1/2 cup sliced black olives
- 1/2 cup diced salami or pepperoni
- 1/2 cup diced provolone cheese
- 1/4 cup sliced pepperoncini peppers
- 2 tbsp red wine vinegar
- 1 tbsp olive oil
- 1 tsp Italian seasoning
- Salt and pepper to taste

Instructions:

1. In a large salad bowl, combine the chopped romaine lettuce, cherry tomatoes, cucumber, red onion, black olives, salami/pepperoni, provolone cheese, and pepperoncini peppers.

2. In a small bowl, whisk together the red wine vinegar, olive oil, and Italian seasoning. Season with salt and pepper.

3. Drizzle the vinaigrette over the salad and toss gently to coat.

4. Serve immediately.

Variations:
- Add cooked and cooled pasta for an Antipasto Pasta Salad
- Swap in different cured meats like prosciutto or capicola
- Use a variety of cheese like mozzarella, parmesan, or asiago
- Add marinated artichoke hearts or roasted red peppers

This Antipasto Salad is a hearty, flavorful salad that makes a great main dish or side. The combination of greens, cured meats, cheese, and tangy vinaigrette creates a delicious Italian•inspired meal. Enjoy!

100. Watermelon feta salad

Ingredient:

- 4 cups cubed seedless watermelon
- 1 cup crumbled feta cheese
- 1/4 cup thinly sliced red onion
- 1/4 cup chopped fresh mint
- 2 tbsp balsamic glaze
- 1 tbsp olive oil
- Juice of 1 lime
- Salt and pepper to taste

Instructions:

1. In a large bowl, gently toss together the cubed watermelon, crumbled feta cheese, sliced red onion, and chopped fresh mint.

2. In a small bowl, whisk together the balsamic glaze, olive oil, and lime juice. Season with a pinch of salt and pepper.

3. Drizzle the dressing over the watermelon salad and toss gently to coat.

4. Serve immediately or refrigerate until ready to serve.

Tips:
- For best flavor, use ripe, juicy watermelon.
- Adjust the amount of feta, onion, and mint to your taste preferences.
- You can substitute balsamic vinegar for the balsamic glaze if desired.
- Add a sprinkle of crushed red pepper flakes for a little kick.

This Watermelon Feta Salad is a refreshing and flavorful summer dish. The sweet watermelon pairs perfectly with the salty feta, tangy lime, and herbaceous mint. It's a light and healthy option that's sure to impress. Enjoy!

101. Roasted vegetables (broccoli, cauliflower, zucchini, etc.)

Ingredient:

• 1 head broccoli, cut into florets
• 1 head cauliflower, cut into florets
• 2 medium zucchini, sliced into 1/2•inch rounds
• 1 red onion, cut into 1•inch wedges
• 3 tbsp olive oil
• 2 tsp dried Italian seasoning
• 1 tsp garlic powder
• Salt and pepper to taste

Instructions:

1. Preheat your oven to 400°F (200°C).

2. In a large bowl, combine the broccoli florets, cauliflower florets, zucchini slices, and red onion wedges.

3. Drizzle the vegetables with the olive oil and sprinkle with the Italian seasoning, garlic powder, salt, and pepper. Toss to coat the vegetables evenly.

4. Spread the seasoned vegetables in a single layer on a large baking sheet lined with parchment paper or a silicone baking mat.

5. Roast the vegetables in the preheated oven for 20•25 minutes, or until they are tender and lightly browned, stirring halfway through.

6. Remove the roasted vegetables from the oven and serve hot.

Variations:
• Add other vegetables like Brussels sprouts, carrots, or bell peppers.
• Sprinkle with grated parmesan cheese or chopped fresh herbs before serving.
• Toss the roasted vegetables with cooked quinoa or brown rice for a more substantial meal.

This simple roasted vegetable dish is a great way to enjoy a variety of healthy, nutrient•dense vegetables. The high•heat roasting brings out the natural sweetness and caramelizes the edges for a delicious, tender result. Enjoy as a side dish or as the base for a plant•based main course.

102. Grilled asparagus

Ingredient:

- 1 lb asparagus, woody ends trimmed
- 1 tbsp olive oil
- 1 tsp lemon zest
- 1 tbsp lemon juice
- 1 garlic clove, minced
- Salt and pepper to taste

Instructions:

1. Preheat your grill or grill pan to medium•high heat.

2. In a large bowl, toss the trimmed asparagus spears with the olive oil, lemon zest, lemon juice, and minced garlic. Season with a pinch of salt and pepper.

3. Arrange the seasoned asparagus in a single layer on the preheated grill. Grill for 5•7 minutes, turning occasionally, until the asparagus is tender•crisp and lightly charred.

4. Transfer the grilled asparagus to a serving plate. Serve immediately.

Nutrition Info (per serving):
Calories: 80
Protein: 5g
Carbs: 5g
Fat: 5g
Fiber: 3g

This grilled asparagus dish is a great option for an endomorph diet. Asparagus is low in calories and carbs but high in fiber, vitamins, and minerals. The lemon and garlic add flavor without added sugar or fat. Grilling the asparagus gives it a delicious smoky char.

Pair this grilled asparagus with a lean protein like grilled chicken or fish for a complete endomorph•friendly meal. Enjoy!

103. Garlic mashed cauliflower

Ingredient:

• 1 large head of cauliflower, cut into florets
• 2 tbsp unsweetened almond milk
• 2 tbsp plain Greek yogurt
• 2 cloves garlic, minced
• 2 tbsp grated Parmesan cheese
• 1 tbsp olive oil
• Salt and pepper to taste

Instructions:

1. In a large pot, bring 1•2 inches of water to a boil. Add the cauliflower florets, cover, and steam for 10•12 minutes, until very tender.

2. Drain the cauliflower and transfer it to a food processor or high•powered blender.

3. Add the almond milk, Greek yogurt, minced garlic, Parmesan cheese, and olive oil. Blend or process until smooth and creamy, scraping down the sides as needed.

4. Season the mashed cauliflower with salt and pepper to taste.

5. Transfer the garlic mashed cauliflower to a serving bowl and serve hot.

Nutrition Info (per serving):
Calories: 100
Protein: 6g
Carbs: 8g
Fat: 6g
Fiber: 3g

This garlic mashed cauliflower is a great low•carb, endomorph•friendly alternative to traditional mashed potatoes. The cauliflower provides fiber and nutrients, while the Greek yogurt and Parmesan add creaminess and protein. The garlic provides flavor without added sugar.

Serve this as a side dish alongside grilled or roasted meats, fish, or poultry for a complete endomorph•friendly meal. Enjoy!

104. Green beans almondine

Ingredient:

• 1 lb fresh green beans, trimmed
• 2 tbsp unsalted butter
• 1/4 cup sliced almonds
• 2 tbsp lemon juice
• 1 tsp lemon zest
• Salt and pepper to taste

Instructions:

1. Bring a large pot of salted water to a boil. Add the trimmed green beans and cook for 5•7 minutes, until tender•crisp. Drain the beans and set aside.

2. In a large skillet, melt the butter over medium heat. Add the sliced almonds and cook, stirring frequently, for 2•3 minutes until the almonds are lightly toasted.

3. Add the cooked green beans to the skillet with the toasted almonds. Drizzle with the lemon juice and sprinkle with the lemon zest. Toss to coat the beans evenly.

4. Season the green beans almondine with salt and pepper to taste.

5. Serve the green beans almondine warm.

Variations:
• For a richer flavor, use browned butter instead of regular butter.
• Add a pinch of garlic powder or red pepper flakes for extra seasoning.
• Sprinkle with grated Parmesan cheese before serving.

Green beans almondine is a classic side dish that pairs well with a variety of main courses. The crunchy toasted almonds and bright lemon flavor complement the tender green beans perfectly. This simple recipe is sure to become a new family favorite!

105. Spaghetti squash

Ingredient:

- 1 medium spaghetti squash, halved lengthwise and seeded
- 1 tbsp olive oil
- Salt and pepper to taste

Instructions:

1. Preheat your oven to 400°F (200°C).

2. Brush the cut sides of the spaghetti squash halves with the olive oil and season with salt and pepper.

3. Place the squash halves cut•side down on a baking sheet lined with parchment paper or a silicone baking mat.

4. Roast the spaghetti squash in the preheated oven for 40•50 minutes, or until the flesh is tender and easily separates into strands when scraped with a fork.

5. Remove the roasted spaghetti squash from the oven and let it cool for 5•10 minutes.

6. Using a fork, gently scrape the flesh of the squash to create long, spaghetti•like strands.

Serving Suggestions:
• Toss the spaghetti squash strands with your favorite pasta sauce, pesto, or sautéed vegetables.
• Top the spaghetti squash with grilled chicken, shrimp, or meatballs for a complete meal.
• Season the spaghetti squash with garlic, herbs, and a drizzle of olive oil or butter.
• Use the spaghetti squash strands as a low•carb alternative to traditional pasta.

Spaghetti squash is a versatile and nutritious vegetable that can be used in a variety of dishes. Roasting brings out its natural sweetness and creates the perfect spaghetti•like texture. Enjoy this healthy and delicious alternative to pasta!

106. Roasted Brussels sprouts

Ingredient:

- 1 lb Brussels sprouts, trimmed and halved
- 2 tbsp olive oil
- 1 tsp garlic powder
- 1 tsp paprika
- 1/4 tsp cayenne pepper (optional)
- Salt and pepper to taste

Instructions:

1. Preheat your oven to 400°F (200°C).

2. In a large bowl, toss the trimmed and halved Brussels sprouts with the olive oil, garlic powder, paprika, and cayenne pepper (if using). Season with a pinch of salt and pepper.

3. Spread the seasoned Brussels sprouts in a single layer on a large baking sheet lined with parchment paper.

4. Roast the Brussels sprouts in the preheated oven for 20•25 minutes, tossing halfway, until they are tender and lightly browned.

5. Remove the roasted Brussels sprouts from the oven and serve hot.

Nutrition Info (per serving):
Calories: 100
Protein: 4g
Carbs: 8g
Fat: 6g
Fiber: 4g

This roasted Brussels sprouts recipe is a great option for an endomorph diet. Brussels sprouts are low in calories and carbs but high in fiber, vitamins, and minerals. The olive oil provides healthy fats, while the garlic powder, paprika, and optional cayenne pepper add flavor without added sugar.

Serve these roasted Brussels sprouts as a side dish to grilled or baked protein sources like chicken, fish, or tofu for a complete endomorph•friendly meal. Enjoy!

107. Stir•fried bok choy

Ingredient:

• 1 lb bok choy, stems and leaves separated and chopped
• 2 tbsp sesame oil
• 2 cloves garlic, minced
• 1 tbsp grated fresh ginger
• 2 tbsp low•sodium soy sauce
• 1 tsp rice vinegar
• 1 tsp sesame seeds (optional)
• Salt and pepper to taste

Instructions:

1. Heat the sesame oil in a large skillet or wok over medium•high heat.

2. Add the chopped bok choy stems and sauté for 2•3 minutes, until they start to soften.

3. Add the minced garlic and grated ginger to the skillet and cook for 1 minute, until fragrant.

4. Add the chopped bok choy leaves and continue to stir•fry for 2•3 minutes, until the leaves are wilted and tender.

5. Drizzle the soy sauce and rice vinegar over the bok choy and toss to coat evenly.

6. Remove the stir•fried bok choy from the heat and sprinkle with sesame seeds, if using.

7. Season with salt and pepper to taste.

8. Serve the stir•fried bok choy hot, as a side dish or over steamed rice or noodles.

Variations:
• Add sliced mushrooms, diced carrots, or other vegetables to the stir•fry.
• Use tamari or coconut aminos instead of soy sauce for a gluten•free option.
• Sprinkle with crushed red pepper flakes for a spicy kick.

Bok choy is a nutrient•dense Chinese cabbage that is delicious when quickly stir•fried. This simple recipe highlights the natural flavors of the bok choy with the addition of garlic, ginger, and a touch of soy sauce. Enjoy this healthy and flavorful side dish!

108. Creamed spinach

Ingredient:

• 1 lb fresh spinach, washed and stems removed
• 1 tbsp olive oil
• 1 clove garlic, minced
• 2 tbsp plain Greek yogurt
• 2 tbsp grated Parmesan cheese
• 1/4 tsp ground nutmeg
• Salt and pepper to taste

Instructions:

1. In a large skillet or saucepan, heat the olive oil over medium heat. Add the minced garlic and cook for 1 minute, until fragrant.

2. Add the fresh spinach to the skillet and cook, stirring frequently, until the spinach is wilted and tender, about 3•5 minutes.

3. Remove the skillet from the heat and let the spinach cool slightly.

4. Transfer the cooked spinach to a food processor or blender. Add the Greek yogurt, Parmesan cheese, and nutmeg. Pulse or blend until the mixture is smooth and creamy.

5. Season the creamed spinach with salt and pepper to taste.

6. Transfer the creamed spinach to a serving bowl and serve warm.

Nutrition Info (per serving):
Calories: 90
Protein: 8g
Carbs: 5g
Fat: 5g
Fiber: 2g

This creamed spinach recipe is a great option for an endomorph diet. Spinach is low in calories and carbs but high in fiber, vitamins, and minerals. The Greek yogurt provides protein and creaminess without the high fat content of traditional cream•based creamed spinach. The Parmesan cheese adds flavor without significantly increasing the carb or fat content.

Serve this creamed spinach as a side dish to grilled or baked protein sources like chicken, fish, or tofu for a complete endomorph•friendly meal. Enjoy!

109. Roasted radishes

Ingredient:

- 1 lb radishes, trimmed and halved
- 1 tbsp olive oil
- 1 tsp dried thyme
- 1/2 tsp garlic powder
- Salt and pepper to taste

Instructions:

1. Preheat your oven to 400°F (200°C).

2. In a large bowl, toss the trimmed and halved radishes with the olive oil, dried thyme, garlic powder, and a pinch of salt and pepper.

3. Spread the seasoned radishes in a single layer on a baking sheet lined with parchment paper.

4. Roast the radishes in the preheated oven for 20•25 minutes, tossing halfway, until they are tender and lightly browned.

5. Remove the roasted radishes from the oven and serve hot.

Nutrition Info (per serving):
Calories: 50
Protein: 1g
Carbs: 5g
Fat: 3g
Fiber: 2g

This roasted radish recipe is a great option for an endomorph diet. Radishes are low in calories and carbs but high in fiber, vitamins, and minerals. The olive oil provides healthy fats, while the thyme and garlic powder add flavor without added sugar.

Roasting brings out the natural sweetness of the radishes and gives them a delicious, crispy texture. Serve these roasted radishes as a side dish to grilled or baked protein sources like chicken, fish, or tofu for a complete endomorph•friendly meal. Enjoy!

110. Sauteed mushrooms

Ingredient:
- 1 lb mixed mushrooms (such as cremini, shiitake, and oyster), sliced
- 1 tbsp olive oil
- 2 cloves garlic, minced
- 1 tbsp fresh thyme leaves (or 1 tsp dried thyme)
- 2 tbsp dry white wine or low·sodium vegetable broth
- Salt and pepper to taste

Instructions:

1. In a large skillet or sauté pan, heat the olive oil over medium·high heat.

2. Add the sliced mushrooms to the pan and sauté for 5·7 minutes, stirring occasionally, until the mushrooms are tender and lightly browned.

3. Add the minced garlic and fresh thyme (or dried thyme) to the pan. Cook for an additional 1·2 minutes, until the garlic is fragrant.

4. Deglaze the pan by pouring in the white wine or vegetable broth. Use a wooden spoon to scrape up any browned bits from the bottom of the pan.

5. Allow the liquid to simmer for 2·3 minutes, until slightly reduced.

6. Season the sautéed mushrooms with salt and pepper to taste.

7. Serve the sautéed mushrooms warm, as a side dish or topping for grilled or roasted proteins.

Nutrition Info (per serving):
Calories: 80
Protein: 3g
Carbs: 5g
Fat: 5g
Fiber: 2g

This sautéed mushroom recipe is a great option for an endomorph diet. Mushrooms are low in calories and carbs but high in fiber, vitamins, and minerals. The olive oil provides healthy fats, while the garlic and thyme add flavor without added sugar.

Enjoy these sautéed mushrooms as a side dish or use them to top grilled chicken, steak, or roasted vegetables for a complete endomorph·friendly meal.

111. Grilled eggplant slices

Ingredient:

- 1 medium eggplant, sliced into 1/2•inch thick rounds
- 2 tbsp olive oil
- 1 tsp dried oregano
- 1 tsp garlic powder
- Salt and pepper to taste

Instructions:

1. Preheat your grill or grill pan to medium•high heat.

2. In a large bowl, toss the eggplant slices with the olive oil, dried oregano, and garlic powder. Season with a pinch of salt and pepper.

3. Arrange the seasoned eggplant slices on the preheated grill or grill pan. Grill for 4•5 minutes per side, or until the eggplant is tender and lightly charred.

4. Transfer the grilled eggplant slices to a serving plate.

Serving Suggestions:
• Serve the grilled eggplant as a side dish, drizzled with a bit of balsamic glaze or lemon juice.
• Top the eggplant slices with crumbled feta cheese, chopped fresh basil, or a dollop of Greek yogurt.
• Use the grilled eggplant slices as a base for a Mediterranean•inspired salad or grain bowl.
• Incorporate the grilled eggplant into a vegetable•based lasagna or moussaka.

Nutrition Info (per serving):
Calories: 80
Protein: 2g
Carbs: 6g
Fat: 6g
Fiber: 3g

This grilled eggplant recipe is a great option for an endomorph diet. Eggplant is low in calories and carbs but high in fiber, vitamins, and antioxidants. The olive oil provides healthy fats, while the oregano and garlic add flavor without added sugar.

Enjoy these versatile grilled eggplant slices as a side dish or incorporate them into a variety of endomorph•friendly meals.

112. Baked zucchini chips

Ingredient:

- 2 medium zucchini, sliced into 1/4•inch thick rounds
- 1 tbsp olive oil
- 1 tsp garlic powder
- 1 tsp paprika
- 1/4 tsp cayenne pepper (optional)
- Salt and pepper to taste

Instructions:

1. Preheat your oven to 400°F (200°C). Line two baking sheets with parchment paper.

2. In a large bowl, toss the zucchini slices with the olive oil, garlic powder, paprika, and cayenne pepper (if using). Season with a pinch of salt and pepper.

3. Arrange the seasoned zucchini slices in a single layer on the prepared baking sheets, making sure they are not overlapping.

4. Bake the zucchini chips in the preheated oven for 12•15 minutes, flipping them halfway through, until they are crispy and lightly browned.

5. Remove the baked zucchini chips from the oven and let them cool for a few minutes before serving.

Nutrition Info (per serving):
Calories: 50
Protein: 2g
Carbs: 4g
Fat: 3g
Fiber: 1g

These baked zucchini chips are a great low•carb, endomorph•friendly snack or side dish. Zucchini is low in calories and carbs but high in fiber, vitamins, and minerals. The olive oil provides healthy fats, while the garlic powder, paprika, and optional cayenne pepper add flavor without added sugar.

Enjoy these crispy baked zucchini chips on their own or pair them with grilled or roasted proteins for a complete endomorph•friendly meal. They also make a great alternative to traditional potato chips.

113. Roasted spaghetti squash

Ingredient:

• 1 medium spaghetti squash, halved lengthwise and seeded
• 1 tbsp olive oil
• 1 tsp dried Italian seasoning
• 1/2 tsp garlic powder
• Salt and pepper to taste

Instructions:

1. Preheat your oven to 400°F (200°C).

2. Brush the cut sides of the spaghetti squash halves with the olive oil. Sprinkle with the dried Italian seasoning, garlic powder, and a pinch of salt and pepper.

3. Place the seasoned spaghetti squash halves cut•side down on a baking sheet lined with parchment paper.

4. Roast the spaghetti squash in the preheated oven for 40•50 minutes, or until the flesh is tender and easily separates into strands when scraped with a fork.

5. Remove the roasted spaghetti squash from the oven and let it cool for 5•10 minutes.

6. Using a fork, gently scrape the flesh of the squash to create long, spaghetti•like strands.

Serving Suggestions:
• Toss the spaghetti squash strands with your favorite endomorph•friendly pasta sauce, such as a simple tomato sauce or pesto.
• Top the roasted spaghetti squash with grilled or baked chicken, shrimp, or tofu for a complete endomorph•friendly meal.
• Season the spaghetti squash with additional herbs, garlic, and a drizzle of olive oil or lemon juice.

This roasted spaghetti squash recipe is a great low•carb, endomorph•friendly alternative to traditional pasta. Spaghetti squash is high in fiber and nutrients but low in calories and carbs, making it an ideal choice for an endomorph diet. The Italian seasoning and garlic add flavor without added sugar or fat.

As you reach the end of "A Comprehensive Body," we hope that you have found inspiration, motivation, and valuable insights to support your fitness journey. Throughout this book, we have provided you with a comprehensive approach to building muscle, incorporating effective exercise plans, and following a 30-day meal plan filled with over 110 delicious recipes for every meal of the day.

By committing to the workout routines, nutritional guidance, and meal options outlined in this book, you have taken a significant step towards achieving your fitness goals and improving your overall health and well-being. Remember that building a strong and healthy body is a journey that requires dedication, consistency, and a positive mindset.

As you continue on your path to a healthier lifestyle, we encourage you to stay focused on your goals, listen to your body, and make adjustments as needed to ensure that you are progressing in a way that is sustainable and fulfilling. Remember that fitness is not just about physical strength; it is also about mental resilience, self-care, and self-improvement.

We believe that with the knowledge and tools provided in "A Comprehensive Body," you have the power to transform your body, enhance your fitness level, and cultivate a positive relationship with exercise and nutrition. Embrace the journey, celebrate your achievements, and always remember that your health and well-being are worth investing in.

Thank you for choosing "A Comprehensive Body" as your guide to building muscle, following effective exercise plans, and nourishing your body with wholesome meals. We wish you continued success on your fitness journey and a lifetime of health and happiness.